The Power Food Cookbook

Energise your life with over 150 simple recipes

Amanda Grant

Photography by David Loftus

For my mummy, who I miss so terribly, and for Ella

A big thank you goes to my gorgeous husband, David, for all his love and support; he is the best taster I know. Special thanks to Vicki, my agent, for encouraging me to write this book and to Rowena, Laura and the team at Hodder, who are just the best to work with. Thanks to David Loftus for, as always, stunning photography. A big thank you to everyone who has helped with the research and recipe testing for the book, including Billy at Books for Cooks, and Katherine.

Photography by David Loftus

Design by Studio Myerscough

First published in Great Britain in 2000 by
Hodder and Stoughton
A division of Hodder Headline

10 9 8 7 6 5 4 3 2 1

A CIP catalogue record for this title is available
from the British Library.

ISBN 0 340 75194 0

Printed and bound in Great Britain by
The Bath Press

Hodder and Stoughton
A division of Hodder Headline
338 Euston Road
London NW1 3BH

Contents

1 *Introduction*

22 *Shopping and ingredients*

36 *Chapter 1: Breakfasts and drinks*

38 *Drinks*

45 *Quick and fruity dishes*

60 *Chapter 2: Mid-morning boosts*

62 *Quick snack ideas*

64 *Warm and fruity*

67 *Cold and fruity*

71 *Bars*

72 *Very quick sandwiches/things on toast*

76 *Chapter 3: Lunches*

78 *Soups*

86 *Warm salads*

91 *Cold salads*

115 *A few sandwiches*

118 *Chapter 4: Mid-afternoon boosts and pre-dinner nibbles*

119 *Very quick mid-afternoon boosts*

120 *Versatile nibbles*

123 *Dips/spreads for vegetable sticks, breads or salads*

127 *Quick hot snacks*

131 *Things to go on bread/toast*

132 *Sweet nibbles*

134 *Chapter 5: Suppers*

136 *Starters or little nibbles*

141 *Main courses*

160 *Chapter 6: Something sweet*

167 *Index*

Introduction

Introduction

Everyone wants and needs more energy. In order to keep pace with the increasing pressures of our lives we need to be more aware of what we eat and the effect food has on our bodies.

First and foremost, *The Power Food Cookbook* is a collection of different ways of combining healthy ingredients. I hope this compilation of recipes will help you to take the steps needed to a healthier way of eating, and eating for energy. Then, you will be on the road to getting the best out of the foods you eat and the best out of life.

Many people complain of a lack of energy and too much stress. The net result is fatigue, tiredness or exhaustion, lethargy, apathy, poor concentration and lack of motivation. To regain a feeling of energy, many people turn to stimulants, for example sugary foods, coffee and cigarettes. But these are unsatisfactory and only lead to short-term energy increases and even more stress. Once you become dependent on the adrenalin kicks from these stimulants, you may also find it harder to relax or sleep when you choose.

The good news, however, is that most people experience a substantial increase in energy within thirty days of improving their diet and significantly reducing their intake of coffee, tea, chocolate and sugary snacks.

Food should smell, taste and look great for it be enjoyable and for us to want to eat it. But food needs to be much more than that. The adage 'you are what you eat' has a lot of truth in it. Our bodies are made up of what we put into them and what we digest and absorb from these foods. We do not need food just to satisfy our hunger, we need it to provide energy and to feed our brains. Would you put poor-quality fuel into your car and expect it to run efficiently?

I studied Food and Nutrition at university and have continued to do so for many years since. Food and nutrition is my real passion. This book is an opportunity to share with you what I have learnt and benefited from. My mother died from cancer. What she and I discovered about nutrition during the last five years of her life made me realise just how important diet can be.

'Diet is an ambiguous tool, too complex and emotionally charged to be prescribed lightly, yet too powerful to be ignored.'
Steven Bradman, MD

Energy is the essence of life, the force that makes everything feasible and achievable. In the body, energy is produced by billions of tiny powerhouses, or cells, and for our bodies to function at peak efficiency we must provide the optimum conditions for each cell to do its work. To achieve this, our bodies need the full range of essential nutrients – fat, carbohydrates, protein, vitamins and minerals – but we also need them to be available in a form in which they can be most readily absorbed.

My message is very simple. Whatever your sex, age or size, if you want to work towards a healthy lifestyle and to have more energy, you need to eat fresh, whole foods. Try to cut out processed, ready-made and high-fat fast foods, and cut right down on caffeine, nicotine and alcohol. Eat a good portion of your food raw and wherever possible choose organic foods.

What foods should we be eating?

The benefits of a traditional diet

Before modern distribution methods, people ate locally grown seasonal food. Those living in a cold northern climate ate foods that were grown in that climate. People had to eat the foods that were in season, which meant that soft fruits and fresh vegetables were more common during the warmer months, while rich warming stews and pickles were eaten during the colder months. In hindsight, this seems like a natural way of adjusting the body to suit the changes in the season.

We ate simple, whole foods creating a diet that was naturally low in fat, high in complex carbohydrates and moderate in protein. Although life and living conditions were hard, people managed to maintain reasonable levels of health despite a lack of modern health care. Looking around the world today, the societies that still retain a traditional approach to diet, such as the Chinese, enjoy the lowest incidence of cancer, heart disease and other degenerative illnesses.

Today, by eating foods from all over the world regardless of the seasons, we have become more dependent on artificial support systems, whether from nutritional supplements, medicines or an artificial environment. Instead we should be making more of an effort to eat locally grown seasonal produce. In order to help you enjoy the benefits of fresh seasonal produce I have included a section on the British Food Calendar on pages 26–27.

The challenges of a modern diet

In the last thirty years, many foods have changed drastically from their natural state due to developments in preserving and packaging. Fresh home-cooked foods have been replaced by pre-cooked, dried, canned, frozen or microwave foods and our daily intake of sugar, meat, processed and refined food has increased. All of these foods, plus quick ready-meals and fast foods, are energy-draining ways to eat. They also present our digestive system with quite a task because they are the most difficult foods to break down.

Our bodies are not equipped to handle the refined flours, sugars, huge quantities of protein and fat that make up our Western fare. Refined high-sugar foods such as cakes, biscuits and chilled desserts are a new invention as far as our digestive system is concerned. Very few naturally occurring foods contain the concentrations of fast-releasing sugars that modern food provides, which make our blood sugar levels rocket and require all sorts of hormones to swing into action to restore balance.

Additives, nuclear irradiation and genetic engineering have also changed the nature of many foods. The further we move into a world of artificial surroundings, processed foods and a sedentary lifestyle, the more stretched is the umbilical cord that connects us to the source of life.

The food we eat is the single greatest influence on our wellbeing. Biology, history and common sense tell us that changes in the food a species lives off will eventually alter it. There are many indications that our diet can be linked to the increase in degenerative illnesses such as cancer and heart disease, and that our diet is not providing us with the energy we need to lead our busy lives.

Go organic

Eating organic may be one answer to many of our health problems, including fatigue, because it provides better nutritional value and no chemicals, pesticides and additives that disrupt our bodies and energy levels (see pages 23–24).

Eat raw

For more energy, we need to increase the amount of raw foods that we eat. Raw energy has been used throughout the civilised world for thousands of years as a way of improving physical health and enhancing awareness. Raw energy principles also form the basis of health and rejuvenation treatment at Europe's and America's finest health farms and spas. Eating foods in this state can enhance cellular vitality, restore a healthy metabolism and put virtually endless energy at our disposal. Indeed, in parts of the world where longevity is taken for granted – by the Hunza tribesmen in the Himalayàs, the Lamas of Tibet and the Fakirs of India – diets are rich in nuts, berries, fruits and fermented milk products, all eaten in their natural 'whole' state, not processed or refined.

There is continuing research about enzymes in food that supports this. All foods contain enzymes and co-factors (vitamins or minerals linked to an enzyme) needed to break down that particular food. If we destroy these enzymes by cooking or processing the foods, then our bodies have to make more of our own digestive enzymes to break down and properly digest food. Without the enzymes from raw foods, our bodies' own enzyme-producing abilities may start to decline. Consequently, over time, we may make fewer enzymes, which limits the effectiveness of our digestive system.

A good way of boosting our enzyme potential is to eat raw foods, which in their natural state contain significant amounts of enzymes. It is also important to chew the foods properly to liberate and activate both the enzymes they contain and our digestive enzymes. A raw food diet can also calm an irritated and overactive digestive system so that its functions can gradually return to normal. Eating more raw foods also helps to reduce our chances of suffering from food sensitivities and chronic digestive disturbances.

Fresh uncooked fruits and vegetables, sprouted seeds and grains also contain higher levels of water than when cooked. This water is found naturally in living cells. Water is invaluable for helping our body to transport nutrients to cells and for taking toxic waste and fat away and enhancing overall vitality. This natural water is very different to the water we drink from a bottle; water in fresh foods carries vitamins, organic minerals, proteins, electrolytes, amino acids, carbohydrates, natural sugars, fatty acids and other nutrients. It helps to create energy and boost cell metabolism.

Phytochemicals

The most recently discovered natural plant substances are known as phytochemicals (*phyto* meaning plant in Greek), which are biologically active compounds in food that interact in complex but complementary ways. Research is showing that they can have a major impact on our lives, helping to promote health and prevent disease. For example, some phytochemicals have been shown to help protect against cancer and certain forms of radiation, to kill germs and act as a powerful wound healer. These phytochemicals have been described as spark plugs for various actions and behaviours within the body's nutritional system and their effect on our health may prove as important as that of vitamins and minerals. Indeed, some scientists are claiming that they can exert unimaginable protective influences on human health.

Cooking food not only destroys enzymes, but it also reduces the activity of phytochemicals. As we do not store phytochemicals in the body it is best to eat foods that can supply us with them so I would stress again the importance of eating fresh fruits and vegetables in their natural state. Research has also revealed that food factors such as antioxidants and phytochemicals work best when they are in food rather than pills. A nutritional supplement or vitamin pill is not as effective as eating the fresh foods, which are absorbed far more easily into the body.

So remember, every time we eat a combination of fresh fruit and vegetables, we are giving ourselves a cocktail of essential vitamins, minerals, amino acids, phytochemicals and enzymes that work together to promote our health.

Top tips:

Have a salad as a major part of one meal every day.

Eat as many foods raw as possible.

Eat a good selection of fresh fruits and vegetables to get a good supply of enzymes, antioxidants and phytochemicals.

Eat organic and seasonal foods.

The way we eat

Today, we spend less time preparing and eating food, and our eating habits have become more casual, with a greater reliance on snacking, takeaways, convenience foods and eating out. When we do eat we choose to do other things at the same time, which is not good news for our digestive system.

The Taylor Nelson Family Food Panel, a body that researches food trends, has proposed six broad types of eating occasion to help to explain our eating habits today:

Snacking: for the winter/spring period of 1997–1998 alone, 17 per cent of all in-home meal occasions were defined as instances of snacking. Those more likely to indulge in this eating behaviour are children and young adults, for some of which snacks are beginning to replace regular meals.

Snatching: today, we are all desperate to make the most of every second of our time, which very often means doing two things at once. Eating has become less of a sociable part of our day and more of an essential incidental. We are eating while doing something else, whether it is shopping, travelling or meeting friends. As a result, very often we are not giving our bodies time to properly digest food.

Cheating in: in the past a woman's worth was measured in terms of her ability to cook nourishing, tasty meals for her family. Nowadays, cheating with a combination of bought and homemade foods has become far more acceptable.

Dining down: this is primarily about convenience, not indulgence. It is a kind of displaced cheating in, focused on budget restaurants. Here, saving time and energy is seen to be worth more than the money spent on the meal.

As well as these issues about when we eat, we are also concerned about the effect of chemical additives in food and confused by the conflicting food messages, whether relating to GM foods, BSE or food allergies.

As we eat out more or snack on the run, it is even more important to make sure that when we do make food at home, it is good for our bodies and quick to prepare. This book contains recipes for meals and snacks that use fresh, seasonal and preferably organic ingredients.

Because of our active and hectic lifestyles, I have written recipe ideas for five meal times during the day to help keep our energy levels high. If we prevent our bodies experiencing long periods between food, we will have less chance to reach a low in energy before a high. Eating small meals often helps to even out blood sugar levels, resulting in more consistent energy, mood and concentration. The mid-morning and mid-afternoon boosts do not need to take long to make – for example, I suggest carrying a bag of organic sunflower seeds, pumpkin seeds or almonds and munching on these when you get hungry in between lunch and supper. Five meals can be sensibly spaced throughout the day; 8.30 a.m. – breakfast; 11 a.m. – first boost; 1.30 p.m. – lunch; 3 p.m. – second boost; 6.30 p.m. – supper. It is important not to eat food late in the evening as this prevents it from being digested effectively and you from having a good night's sleep. When you eat away from home, try to be more discerning about the foods you choose to eat. Finally, we must also make a concerted effort to give our bodies enough time to digest the foods that we eat.

How we make use of the food that we eat

Without proper digestion, there can be no such thing as good nutrition. The effectiveness of our digestion determines our energy level, longevity and state of mind and body. A lack of nutrients and eating the wrong kind of food can result in faulty digestion, faulty absorption, abnormal gut reactions including bloating and inflammation, infections and poor elimination. The knock-on effects disrupt every body system: our immunity, the brain and nervous system, hormonal balance and our ability to detoxify.

Our bodies use more energy on the digestion of food than on almost any other function. This is why we can feel lethargic and lacking in energy after a big meal. Our bodies have had to redirect blood (and therefore energy) away from the brain and other organs towards the gut. This enables the body to break down the food we have eaten and transform it into chemicals, which can be absorbed in the bloodstream and then our cells. There it is turned into the building blocks of life; energy needed both physically and mentally.

One of our body's prime functions is to eliminate food wastes from our systems. These would otherwise accumulate and decay in our colon, breeding bacteria that release toxins which get into the bloodstream, spreading all sorts of sickness throughout the body. In a healthy body, the residues of digested food pass through the small intestine into the colon in liquid form and are eventually eliminated from the bowels. The fibres in raw foods assist this process, acting as a kind of intestinal broom. However, with processed food, the action becomes more like a filthy mop that leaves a trail of sludge coating the intestinal walls, which can make the colon sluggish and slow.

We need to have a brief understanding of how our digestive system works in order to make informed choices about the combination of foods to eat and the best times to eat them.

Digestion

The digestive system breaks down food and readies it for absorption. This process begins with the senses. The sight and smell of food initiate chemical reactions that get us ready to digest foods. Chewing is particularly important because messages are sent to the digestive tract to prepare different enzyme secretions according to what is in the mouth. These digestive enzymes are essential to break down the foods we eat into usable nutrients. A healthy body produces thousands of enzymes, each of which has a specific job: protein is broken down into amino acids, complex carbohydrates into simple sugars, fat into fatty acids and glycerol. Every day ten litres of digestive juices, mostly produced by the pancreas, liver, stomach and intestinal wall, pour into the digestive tract. For the body to make these enzymes it needs nutrients. If we do not absorb sufficient nutrients, digestion is not as effective as it should be, which in turn can create a situation where poor absorption and nutritional intake gets progressively worse.

Similarly, crash dieting, poor eating or stress all lead to enzyme depletion because the body is deprived of the nutrients it needs and food may not break down properly. This can result in a lowering of energy after we have eaten, or the kind of digestive disturbance that causes feelings of hunger after a meal and triggers overeating. If we can work towards improving our digestion, research shows that energy levels can improve.

Acid and alkaline-forming foods

Once food has been broken down in the mouth, it moves on to the stomach where large proteins are broken down into smaller groups called amino acids. The stomach produces a range of enzymes, collectively called proteases, to break down this protein.

The type of food we eat will affect the internal environment of our stomach, intestines and bowels. Common acid-forming foods include coffee, sugar, citrus fruits and wine. They create a condition in our stomach that can lead to indigestion. The body needs a certain amount of acid, but when there is too much, problems can arise. Foods such as meat create a more acidic condition because they require us to secrete stronger acids to aid digestion. Stress also makes our body secrete more acid into the digestive system, which accounts for the gnawing feeling in our stomach when we are tense. As the acids are absorbed, our blood normally becomes more acidic, but if the blood is already acidic, various health problems can arise, including indigestion, headaches, cystitis and difficulty in relaxing. And if over-acidity is allowed to persist,we can be more predisposed to rheumatoid arthritis, stomach ulcers and cancer.

Reducing the amount of acid-forming foods in our diet can help to reduce the acidity of our blood. Increasing the quantity of grains, vegetables and beans can help to make our blood more alkaline and therefore counter-balance too much acidity. Roughly 80 per cent of our diet should come from alkaline-forming foods and 20 per cent from acid-forming foods.

Examples of high acid-forming foods include:
bacon, beef, chicken, eggs, fish and shellfish

Those that are medium acid-forming foods include:
herrings, mackerel, wheat, rice, plums, Brazil nuts

High alkaline-forming foods include: avocado, beetroot, carrots, spinach, potatoes, dried fruits, rhubarb

Medium alkaline-forming foods include:
apricots, apples, banana, berries, cherries, figs, grapefruit, beans, cabbage, mushrooms, onions, root vegetables, tomatoes, celery

Protein is digested in the first part of the small intestine, the duodenum, into which flow digestive enzymes produced in the pancreas and liver. The pancreas is the primary organ of digestion. The enzymes it produces for breaking down carbohydrates, fats and proteins are called amylase, lipase and proteases.

Fat has to be specially prepared before being digested. This is achieved by a substance called bile, produced by the liver and stored in the gall bladder. Bile contains lecithin, which helps to emulsify large fat particles and turns them into tiny particles with a greater surface area for the fat-splitting lipase enzyme to work on.

A diet high in saturated fats, such as meat, eggs and cheese, will tend to slow down food moving through your digestive system. It usually takes high fibre foods between twelve and twenty-four hours to pass through your intestines, but meat typically takes forty-eight hours. And in an elderly person, it can take up to two weeks.

Food Combining

Many people have found that certain food combinations do not suit them. Based on this observation and his research into health and nutrition, Dr Howard Hay devised a diet plan popularly known as 'food combining'. This diet plan has helped millions of people towards better health. Hundreds of years of conventional and complementary medical experience has shown that eating a diet high in raw ingredients and also avoiding certain combinations of foods aids digestion and detoxification. Food combining lies at the basis of virtually every tradition of natural healing.

In his diet plan, Dr Hay formulated rules about which foods you can eat together. In the original theory, the key elements were to eat alkaline-forming foods, avoid refined and heavily processed foods, eat fruit on its own and to eat protein-rich foods and carbohydrate-rich foods separately.

Food combining is not something that we should become neurotic about. Some people with strong digestive systems seem to be able to mix any healthy foods together and still feel full of energy. However, if you suffer from weight gain or poor indigestion, thinking about your foods and how to combine them may be a blessing.

Eat fruit on its own Fruit is one of the best fuels for instant energy, requiring very little digestion. Many kinds of soft fruits ferment rapidly once ripe. They will do the same if we put them in a warm, acidic environment, like the stomach. Fruit is digested incredibly quickly, sometimes remaining in the stomach for as little as fifteen to twenty minutes. However, if we eat fruit at a meal with other foods it may be forced to remain in the stomach for two or more hours and during this time the fruit can start to ferment, which may cause indigestion and wind. If we want to eat fruit with a meal it is best to have it as a starter and to leave twenty minutes before the next course.

So Dr Hay's advice about eating fruit separately from other foods makes a great deal of sense. The best time to eat fruit is as a snack at least thirty minutes before a meal or not less than two hours after a meal. Alternatively, you can combine fruits that do not readily ferment (bananas, apples or coconuts) with complex carbohydrate foods.

The effect of food on our bodies

During digestion the body breaks down the food we eat and transforms it into chemicals, which are absorbed into the bloodstream for use by our cells. Consequently, the food we eat affects the conditions of our organs as the blood travels through them. There has been much research looking at the effects of diet on our bodies and in particular on specific organs.

For example, the liver performs the extremely important function of breaking down unwanted toxic wastes in the body. However, if the wrong sorts of drink and food are continually eaten, it is put under a constant strain because of having to recycle more waste than it can manage, and can become overloaded. The toxins, which should be expelled from the body, and the majority of which are fat soluble, are then taken by the blood and lymph to be stored in cells as fat.

The heart is another organ directly effected by our diet. Blood that is rich in fats increases the risk of hardened, clogged arteries, which strain the heart, leading in extreme cases to coronary heart disease. It is now thought that with appropriate exercise and a diet with less than 10 per cent fat this process can be reversed. This is borne out by WHO research, which has found that British vegetarians have a 30 per cent lower rate of coronary heart disease.

It has been found that women whose diet is high in fats and protein reach menopause at an average age of fifty, whereas those who eat little or no animal fats begin at an average age of forty-six. The later menopause starts, the greater the risk of breast cancer.

To diminish the risk of stroke and coronary heart disease we should eat a diet low in fat and high in complex carbohydrates, found in grains, vegetables and beans. In addition, reduce your intake of alcohol and salt and do not be fooled by low-fat alternatives: these have been shown to be just as harmful as traditional sources of saturated fat. It is not clear that eating margarine is any healthier than butter. It is best to use olive oil or a spread made from pure olive oil or products such as tahini.

Top tips:

Eat 80 per cent alkaline-forming foods, 20 per cent acid-forming foods and eat large quantities of vegetables and fruit. Eat good sources of concentrated protein foods such as beans, lentils and whole grains rather than lots of meat, fish, cheese and eggs. See lists of acid- and alkaline-forming foods on page 7.

Eat fast fermenting (most soft fruits, including peaches, plums, mangoes, papayas, strawberries and melon) and acid fruits (oranges, lemons, grapefruit and pineapple) on their own as snacks. All of these fruits require little digestion, releasing their natural fructose content quickly.

Eat concentrated proteins and concentrated carbohydrates separately. For example, eat animal or fish proteins with vegetables instead of carbohydrates.

High-protein foods take a long time to digest fully, therefore they help to stabilise blood-sugar swings and help to maintain energy levels.

Avoid refined carbohydrates such as white sugar, white bread, processed cakes and biscuits. Eat unrefined, fast-releasing carbohydrates with unrefined slow-releasing carbohydrates such as bananas, apples and coconut, which can be combined with slow-releasing carbohydrates such as oats and millet; or eat potatoes, rice or bread with root vegetables, salad vegetables and chickpeas; eat apples, bananas or coconuts with oats or wheat.

How we use energy to live

Without energy the body cannot function, at work, rest or play. Energy, or to be specific, chemical energy, fuels our body processes such as metabolism and body temperature. Once food is eaten, chemical reactions break proteins, fats, carbohydrates and alcohol down into glucose, which drives the body.

Reduced to a simple equation:

glucose + oxygen = carbon dioxide (which we exhale), water (some of which we excrete) and energy.

Metabolic rate is the speed at which your body processes the food you eat into energy and bodily structures.

It is made up of two inter-related factors:

Basal metabolic rate (BMR) – the energy it takes just to exist, i.e., the energy it takes to keep your heart beating, lungs breathing and your other vital internal functions.

Resting metabolic rate (RMR) – this includes the BMR plus additional energy expenditures required for activity. Your RMR accounts for approximately 60 per cent of the energy you expend daily. The higher this rate the more efficient your body is at burning fat.

It is the RMR that slows down when you restrict calories. In a one year study of overweight men, those who cut calories to lose weight, as opposed to those who exercised, experienced a significant drop in their RMR (RMR is closely linked to how much muscle you have). This helps to explain why 95 to 99 per cent of people who crash diet are likely to regain their weight, with interest, within a year.

The different sources of energy

It is not essential to be too concerned about exact quantities of protein, carbohydrate etc. that you should be eating a day. However, it is a good idea to have a general understanding of nutrients and the main foods in which they can be found. We get our energy from a mixture of nutrients (carbohydrates, protein, fat etc.) so it is important that we eat a good balance of these.

Carbohydrates

Carbohydrates break down into glucose, which is the fuel for our muscles, brain and central nervous system. Glucose is the body's primary energy source and it therefore makes sense that carbohydrates should make up the major part of our diet.

The energy in food is measured in calories and carbohydrates provide four calories per gram. Carbohydrates should account for two-thirds of the calories we consume. Excess carbohydrate is stored in the liver and muscles as glycogen, to be called up when needed as a reserve energy source. If it is not required, it is deposited as fat.

The type of carbohydrate we eat is as important as the amount Carbohydrate comes in two forms: 'fast-releasing' or simple carbohydrates, such as sugar, honey, sweets and most refined products (products which more often than not have been stripped of their natural fibre, most of their minerals, vitamins and trace elements); and 'slow-releasing' or complex carbohydrates including whole grains, vegetables and fresh fruits.

Fast-releasing carbohydrates are absorbed very quickly into our bloodstream, upsetting the pancreas and disrupting the steady flow of energy in your body. This helps to explain why very often, sugary snacks will give us an instant high followed straightaway by a low. Foods containing refined sugars, such as sweets, cakes and convenience foods, place more extreme demands on your body. If sugary foods are eaten throughout the day, blood sugar levels are likely to seesaw, leading to mood swings and changes in our energy levels. In extreme cases, people become tired, shaky and irritable as their blood sugar reaches its lowest point, which will sabotage any attempt at wellbeing. Worse, over time, this process can have an adverse effect on your pancreas, eventually leading to diabetes.

Very few naturally occurring foods contain the kind of concentrations of fast-releasing sugars as processed foods, and the body is simply not adapted to deal with them. They make your blood sugar levels rocket, requiring all sort of hormones to swing into emergency action to restore the balance, but also feed undesirable micro-organisms that can occur in the gut. The few foods that are good unrefined fast-releasing carbohydrates include bananas, dates and raisins, but these will not make the blood sugar levels seesaw in the same way.

The sort of carbohydrate we need to give us a high level of energy that will last, are the 'slow-releasing' or complex carbohydrates. These are found in whole grains, brown rice, vegetables, fruits and whole grain breads, all of which come as nature intended, complete with natural fibre, essential fatty acids and important vitamins and minerals. Complex carbohydrates take a while to absorb into the system and as a result they provide a steady stream of energy in the form of glucose throughout the day. Ideally, these slow-releasing carbohydrates should make up around 70 per cent of your diet.

Top tips:

Aim to eat three or more daily servings of a variety of fresh fruit such as apples, pears, bananas, berries, melons or citrus fruits.

Eat three or more daily servings of dark green leafy and root vegetables, such as watercress, carrots, sweet potatoes, broccoli, Brussels sprouts, spinach, green beans or peppers, raw or lightly cooked.

Eat three or more daily servings of whole grains such as rice, oats, whole wheat, corn, pasta or pulses.

Fibre

Fibre absorbs water in the digestive tract, making the food contents bulkier and easier to pass through the body. In Britain the average intake of fibre is 22 g a day compared to rural Africans who eat 55 g a day. The Africans have the lowest incidence of bowel diseases such as appendicitis, diverticulitis, colitis and bowel cancer. The ideal intake is not less than 35 g a day and it is easy to eat this amount if we eat whole grains, vegetables, fruits, nuts, seeds, lentils and beans on a daily basis, although cooking decreases the fibre content of food. Fruit and vegetable fibre helps to slow down the absorption of sugar into the blood, helping to maintain good energy levels.

Cereal fibre is particularly good at preventing constipation. See the following suggestions to make it easier to incorporate fibre in your diet:

- oats: see muesli recipes plus others in the Breakfasts chapter
- sunflower seeds: sprinkle over salads (see Lunches) or nibble as a mid-morning snack
- large baked potato with skin on: see Mid-afternoon boosts for dips and topping ideas to go on the jackets
- 3 oranges: see Breakfast drinks and Lunches
- cooked lentils: see Lunches and Suppers
- 3 carrots: see Lunches
- 3 bananas: see Breakfasts and Mid-morning boosts

Protein

Protein is vital for growth and the repair of body tissue. It is also needed to make hormones, enzymes, antibodies and neurotransmitters and it helps to transport substances around the body.

Protein is created in the body by building blocks called amino acids. Many of these amino acids can be manufactured in the body, but some so-called essential amino acids must be obtained from food. Both the quality of the protein we eat and the quantity are important. The best-quality protein foods in terms of amino acid balance include eggs, soya, meat, fish, beans and lentils.

Animal protein sources on the whole tend also to include saturated fats that are not so desirable. However, vegetable protein sources, which include peas, broccoli, corn and runner beans, tend to contain additional beneficial complex carbohydrates and are less acid-forming than meat (see page 7 for acid- and alkaline-forming foods).

Every natural food needs protein to grow, hence if you eat a varied diet with regular meals, it is almost impossible not to get enough protein. The World Health Organisation recommends a minimum intake of 32 g of protein per day, or 4.5 per cent of the calorific value.

The following quantity of protein foods will provide you with 20 g of protein. The first group is classed as 'excellent-quality' protein foods. I have also suggested where to look for recipes that contain these foods to make it easier for you to incorporate them into your diet. As you can see, you do not need to eat vast quantities of these foods so it is easy to eat 32 g of protein a day without too much effort:

- brown rice (400 g/14 oz): see Suppers
- canned tuna (84 g/3½ oz tin): see Lunches
- sardines (100 g/3½ oz tin): see Lunches
- eggs (2 medium): see Breakfasts and Mid-afternoon boosts
- yogurt (450 g/1 lb): see Breakfasts
- tofu (275 g/10 oz)

For 'reasonable-quality' protein foods you need to eat the following amounts of each food to obtain 20 g of protein:

- chickpeas (110 g/ 4 oz): see Lunches and Mid-afternoon boosts
- sunflower seeds (188 g/6½ oz): see Mid-morning boosts and Lunches
- cashew nuts (110 g/4 oz) and almonds (110 g/4 oz): both of these feature in many recipes including Mid-morning boosts and Breakfasts
- spinach (390 g/14 oz): see Lunches and Suppers
- wheat germ (132 g/5 oz): see Breakfasts

Top tips:

Eat two daily servings of beans, lentils, tofu, 'seed' vegetables (such as peas, broad beans) or other vegetable protein.

Eat meat, fish, eggs and cheese in moderation.

Fat

Contrary to popular belief, fat is necessary in the diet and in the right quantities it can be good for us. Fat is a critical component of cell membranes and hormones and is essential in some processes for nutrients to be absorbed into the system. Fat also cushions organs and helps regulate the body temperature by insulating the body. It also yields energy. The types of oils and fats we eat are important if we want to benefit from endless energy.

Oils and fats come in two basic forms, saturated fats and unsaturated fats. Saturated fats are found in animal products such as butter and meat. Unsaturated fats come in two forms, monounsaturated (for example, extra virgin olive oil) and polyunsaturated, found in nut and seed oils (for example, corn oil, groundnut oil, sunflower oil and safflower). Certain polyunsaturated fats called linoleic and linolenic acid or omega 6 and omega 3 oils are vital for the brain and nervous system, immune system and cardiovascular system and skin. If we are deficient in these substances, a common sign is dry skin. Most authorities now agree that no more than one-third of our total fat intake should be saturated and at least one-third should be polyunsaturated.

Experiments have shown that when someone eats a meal high in any kind of fat, the fats form a film around red blood cells and platelets and encourage them to stick together or clump. This clumping causes small capillaries to clog and even shut down so that as much as 20 per cent of our normal blood circulation is lost, reducing the amount of oxygen available to our cells by about 30 per cent. This clumping and its corresponding oxygen-cell deficit lasts for many hours after eating a meal high in fat. The action of fat on the brain is one of the main reasons why we can feel sleepy or unable to think clearly after eating a heavy meal. Fats to avoid are the processed unsaturated fats found in cooking oils, margarine and convenience foods. Instead, get your fats as they come in nature – in whole grains, pulses, nuts, seeds and avocados. Try not to use butter on your toast; if you need a spread try 'only olive', which is made from pure olive oil.

Top tips:

Try to include pumpkin and flaxseeds in the diet, as both are rich in linolenic acid (omega 3).

Sunflower seeds and sesame seeds are rich in linoleic acid (omega 6).

Avoid fats such as shortenings, refined oils and dairy products.

Good sources of natural polyunsaturated oils include fresh fish, such as mackerel, herring, sardines, anchovies and wild trout.

Water

Two-thirds of the human body consists of water and is our most important nutrient. The body loses 1.5 litres (2¾ pints) of water a day through skin, lungs, gut and via the kidneys as urine, ensuring that toxic substances are eliminated from the body. We also make about a third of a litre of water a day when glucose is burnt for energy. Therefore, our minimum intake of water a day needs to be 1 litre (1¾ pints). Ideally, we should aim to drink 2 litres (3½ pints). Fruit and vegetables consist of around 90 per cent water and they supply it in a form that is very easy for the body to use while at the same time providing the body with a high percentage of its vitamins and minerals.

Dehydration can leave us feeling weak and tired and it can lead to overeating, because it disturbs our appetite mechanisms so that we think we are hungry even when we are not. Drinking plenty of pure, clean water detoxifies the body steadily and can help us break the junk food habit. Thoughts and feelings become distorted when our body gets even mildly dehydrated. Research with athletes at Harvard University and Loma Linda University in the United States has demonstrated that drinking extra water reduces fatigue and stress and increases stamina and energy to a remarkable degree. It also eliminates false hunger. Yet few of us drink enough.

On average, in a temperate climate – not sweating from exertion or heat – we need about 3.6 litres/6 pints a day for optimal health, although few of us consume even as much as 1.2 litres/2 pints. Provided you are not suffering from a kidney or liver disease, this needs to be drunk as pure water, not as coffee or tea which are diuretics andcan help the body to lose water that it needs. However, remember that if you consume too much liquid, you can overwork your kidneys and increase your risk of fluid retention.

Top tips:

Keep a bottle of water with you everywhere you go and drink juices and herbal teas.

Alcohol, tea and coffee cause the body to lose water, so are not recommended as sources of fluid intake.

Minerals

Like vitamins, minerals are essential for most body processes. Oxygen is carried in the blood by an iron compound, and a lack of this mineral can lead to anaemia and fatigue. Calcium, magnesium and phosphorus help to form the bones and teeth; and nerve signals, vital for the brain and muscles, depend upon calcium, magnesium, sodium and potassium. These are just a sample of the thousands of key roles that minerals play in human health.

The old school of thought was that people need to eat meat for protein and iron and milk for calcium, but this is not necessarily true. If we take a quick look at some of the main minerals, we can see that there are in fact, many other better food sources for each of these minerals, which will help to provide us with endless energy.

Iron transports oxygen and carbon dioxide to and from cells and it is absolutely vital for energy production. Without sufficient iron in our diet we can experience anaemia, which may lead to fatigue, loss of appetite, nausea and sensitivity to the cold. It is particularly important for pregnant women to make sure their intake of iron is high. There are many sources of iron, including fruits, vegetables, seeds and pulses. It is also worth noting that vitamin C helps iron absorption, so a combination of iron rich and vitamin C rich foods is a good idea.

Good food sources: pumpkin seeds, almonds, prunes, cashew nuts, raisins, brazil nuts, walnuts, dried apricots, cooked dried beans and lentils, sesame seeds, pecan nuts, broccoli, beans, dark green leafy vegetables, peas

Potassium helps to produce secretions of insulin for blood sugar control to produce constant energy. It is vital for the normal balance of water in the body and essential in the production of enzymes, which stimulate energy production. Potassium enables nutrients to move into cells and waste products to move out of cells. It helps to promote healthy nerves and muscles, relaxes muscles and is also involved in metabolism, maintaining heart functioning and stimulating the gut movements to help encourage proper elimination.

If we become deficient in potassium we may experience muscle weakness, pins and needles, cellulite and nausea. Magnesium helps to hold potassium in cells. Excess sodium from salt, alcohol, sugar and stress can help to deplete the supply of potassium.

Good food sources: wholemeal bread, bananas, eggs, nuts, fresh and dried fruits (see Breakfasts), watercress (see Lunches), radishes (see Suppers), mushrooms (see Lunches and Suppers), pumpkin

Zinc is essential for constant energy. It is a component of over two hundred enzymes, and is essential for growth, important for healing, aids the ability to cope with stress effectively and promotes a healthy nervous system and brain, especially in a growing foetus. Zinc also helps in bone and teeth formation and makes, hair look glossy and thick.

If we become deficient in zinc we may experience white marks on our fingernails, acne or greasy skin, loss of appetite and a tendency for depression. Vitamins A, E and B6 as well as magnesium, calcium and phosphorous all help the body to absorb zinc.

Stress, alcohol and a low protein intake can prevent its uptake.

Good food sources: eggs, pecan nuts, brazil nuts, oats, peanuts, almonds, whole wheat grain (see Breakfasts and Mid-morning boosts), lentils, green peas and ginger (see Lunches and Suppers), sesame seeds, sunflower, pine nuts and pumpkin seeds

Calcium helps with bone formation, the prevention of osteoporosis and proper functioning of the heart, muscles and nerves. It also helps to improve skin and teeth health and maintains the correct acid-alkaline balance. If we become deficient in calcium, we may experience high blood pressure, tooth decay or insomnia. Alcohol, lack of exercise and caffeine all inhibit its absorption. Vitamin C and D intake aid its absorption.

Good food sources: brazil nuts, chickpeas, dried seaweed, cheddar cheese, brewer's yeast, yogurt, corn tortillas (see Suppers), globe artichokes, prunes, figs and pumpkin seeds (see Breakfasts), cooked dried beans (see Lunches). Vitamin D and exercise help the body absorb calcium.

Calcium and magnesium are found in vegetables such as kale, cabbage and root vegetables. They are also abundant in nuts and seeds.

Selenium is a powerful antioxidant that protects against heart disease, prostate cancer and lung cancer.

Good food sources: dried mushrooms, sardines, lentils, tuna, wholemeal bread, sunflower seeds, white fish

Top tip:

Eat at least one serving of mineral-rich foods each day. For example: eat a live yogurt for breakfast, fresh kale or root vegetables for supper or have a handful of nuts and seeds for a snack or a bowl of lentil soup for lunch, plus plenty of fresh fruits and vegetables. You will find lots of recipe ideas in each chapter.

Vitamins

Vitamins are vital to us. They 'turn on' enzymes, which in turn help to make the body processes happen. We need vitamins to produce energy, to balance hormones, boost the immune system, make healthy skin and protect arteries. They are also vital for the brain and nervous system. The B and C vitamins are necessary for turning food into energy, both mental and physical. Vitamins A, C and E are all antioxidant vitamins that help to protect us from cancer and help to slow down the ageing process and protect the body from heart disease and pollution. Vitamin D helps to control calcium intake.

Vitamin and mineral supplements

There is no doubt that vitamin and mineral supplements have a valuable role to play both in the prevention and treatment of a wide variety of health problems. However, what we get from pills is a substance that has been artificially manufactured, often with a higher potency than is necessary for good health. There is growing evidence that naturally derived vitamins are more effective than those that are synthetically manufactured, since they are purer in origin and, in many cases, more easily absorbed by the body. Many experts in the complementary field of medicine are advising that the best course of action to take for a healthy lifestyle is to ensure that we get an adequate supply of all essential nutrients from our food.

Below I take a quick look at a few key vitamins, their functions and their food sources. You will also see recommended chapters for recipe ideas using foods that contain these minerals.

Vitamin B1 (thiamine) All of the B vitamins are important in their own ways; vitamin B6 and zinc help insulin to work; vitamin B3 and chromium, plus vitamins B1, B2, B3, B5, co-enzyme Q, (plus vitamin C, iron, copper and magnesium) are all nutrients required to turn glucose within cells into energy. Vitamin B is also required for muscle and nerve transmission, the final process in turning fuel into energy.

Vitamin B1 is essential for energy production, brain function and digestion. This vitamin helps the body to make use of protein and to convert starchy foods into energy. Consequently, lethargy, fatigue, weakness and mood swings are classic symptoms of deficiency in this and many of the other B vitamins.

Studies have shown that thiamine deficiency can cause fatigue, sleeplessness, depression, irritability, difficulty in concentrating, inefficiency and forgetfulness. In more extreme cases, it can lead to certain more severe physical symptoms, including shortness of breath, anaemia and low blood pressure. In the Western world, it is likely that heavy drinkers are the people who are most likely to suffer from thiamine deficiency.

Good food sources: watercress, peppers, cauliflower, cabbage, tomatoes, asparagus, Brussels sprouts, wheat germ, yeast extracts

B2 (riboflavin) converts fats and proteins to energy.

Good food sources: brewer's yeast, cheese, eggs, green leafy vegetables, liver, meat, soya products, wheat germ, yeast extracts, yogurts

B3 (niacin) is needed for brain and nerve function, healthy skin, tongue and digestive organs.

Good food sources: brewer's yeast, cheese, dried fruits, eggs, nuts, oily fish, pig's liver, poultry, whole grain cereals, yeast extracts

B6 (pyridoxine) is needed for protein conversion, protection against heart disease, regulation of menstrual cycle, growth, nervous and immune systems.

Good food sources: bananas, brewer's yeast, cod, lentils, poultry, salmon, wheat germ, walnuts

B12 is needed for metabolism, nervous system, prevention of pernicious anaemia and proper formation of blood cells. With B6, it controls levels of homocysteine, which may cause heart disease.

Good food sources: cheese, eggs, lamb, liver, oily fish, seaweed

Vitamin C strengthens the immune system and helps to fight infections. It also makes collagen, keeping bones, skin and joints firm and strong. This vitamin helps to turn food into energy and makes anti-stress hormones. If you become deficient in vitamin C you may suffer from lack of energy, colds, bleeding or tender gums and slow wound healing. Vitamin C works with the B vitamins to produce energy and it works with vitamin E as an antioxidant. Avoid smoking, stress and fried foods to prevent it from being absorbed and used by the body.

Good food sources: peppers, watercress, cabbage, cauliflower, strawberries, oranges, grapefruit, tomatoes

Vitamin A (retinol) is found in animal form in meat, fish, eggs and dairy produce. Good food sources include lamb's liver (see Lunches), mackerel, salmon and cod.

Vegetable foods, which contain beta-carotene, can be converted by the body to retinol and are therefore a source of vitamin A.

Beta-carotene is an antioxidant that is essential for protection against heart disease, cancer and as an immune-booster. It is also needed for healthy skin and hair and is essential for night vision. Vitamins C and E help to protect the vitamin, whereas wheat, coffee and alcohol all destroy it.

It is found in yellow, orange and green fruits and vegetables.

Good food sources: apricots, chard, dark green and red leaf lettuce, dark leafy greens, mangoes, carrots, pumpkin, spinach, sweet potatoes, watercress, squash

Vitamin E, an antioxidant, is needed to help the body use oxygen, prevent the blood from forming blood clots and improve healing of wounds. It is also good for the skin. If you experience exhaustion after light exercise, easy bruising, slow wound healing, loss of muscle tone or infertility, these may be a result of a lack of this vitamin. Avoid an excessive intake of refined or processed fats and oils.

Good food sources: sunflower seeds, peanuts, wheat germ, sesame seeds, avocado, spinach, tuna, sardines, salmon, sweet potatoes

Folic acid is critical during pregnancy for development of the foetus' brain and nerves but throughout our lives we always need folic acid for brain and nerve functioning. Folic acid is also needed for utilising protein and red blood cell formation. If we become deficient in folic acid we may experience a lack of energy, anaemia, poor appetite, stomach pains and depression.

Good food sources: wheat germ, sesame seeds, cashew nuts, asparagus, broccoli, avocado

Vitamin D helps to maintain strong and healthy bones by retaining calcium. Vitamins A, C and E help to protect vitamin D. Fried foods and a lack of sunlight steal the vitamin away.

Good food sources: canned sardines, herrings, mackerel, salmon, eggs, kippers

Top tips:

Eat three or more servings of fresh fruits, plus seeds or nuts, each day.

Eat three or more servings of dark green, leafy and root vegetables every day.

Seaweed provides an excellent source of vitamins A, C, D, E and K, plus B vitamins, including B12, a vitamin that is rarely present in land vegetables.

Adapting our diet to our activity levels

We should be aware of the link between our activity levels and our food consumption. The more active our jobs or lifestyles, the more energy we require. We also need energy in different forms to compensate for our activity; sometimes we need fast-acting energy, other times it needs to be slow-releasing. We need to match our food intake to our natural biorhythms and lifestyle demands. For instance, people who exercise in the morning without having anything to eat first can feel enormously tired later in the morning. Sports players who do not eat before a match often run into difficulties. Changing the timing of meals can help your body to respond to your lifestyle.

According to sports nutrition research, if we want to improve our physical performance, we must ensure we are giving our body the right fuel. During sustained 'less strenuous' exercise such as jogging, swimming, tennis and walking, carbohydrates yield twice as much energy as fat. Carbohydrates, not fat, are therefore the premier fuel for performance.

Also, carbohydrates can be stored as glycogen, while fat cannot. Glycogen is a short-term store of energy, held in muscles and the liver, and can be used during extended physical performance. For this reason, many athletes eat complex carbohydrates such as bread, pasta and rice a number of hours before their event so that it has time to turn into glycogen.

As a very general guide, if we are active, we need to make sure that we eat plenty of complex carbohydrates (whole grains, fruit, vegetables, beans and lentils, see page 11) and 'load up' before exercising. Avoid eating too much protein and drink plenty of water before and, when possible, during exercise.

Power Food basics

If you are looking for a healthy lifestyle and want to maximise your energy, think about the following:

- Eat small meals frequently – five meals are better than three – carry sunflower seeds, pumpkin seeds, almonds and munch on these when you get hungry as a small meal in between lunch and supper.
- Eat when you are hungry, not out of habit. Graze rather than gorge, small snacks in between meals will help keep your blood sugar levels even and energy levels constant.
- Sit and eat your food calmly without doing something else at the same time.
- Eat a varied diet using whole foods grown on healthy soils, simply prepared and eaten as close to their natural state as possible; for example, eat the skin of potatoes and the germ and bran of wheat.
- Eat vegetables, fruit, sprouted seeds, fish, whole grains (barley, rice, pulses), nuts and a little meat. A diet containing these foods is low in saturated fats and refined sugars, moderate in protein and high in fibre and complex carbohydrates.
- Eat unrefined, slow-releasing carbohydrates (whole grain cereals, pasta, breads), which release their fuel slowly, a couple of times a day. For fast energy eat these with unrefined fast-releasing carbohydrates. For example, fruits such as bananas, apples and coconut, can be combined with slow-releasing carbohydrate cereals like oats and millet. Avoid refined carbohydrates.
- Ensure that you have optimum intakes of all essential nutrients (vitamins, minerals etc.).
- Avoid stimulants and depressants (coffee, tea, cigarettes etc.) as much as possible and limit your alcohol intake.
- Eat a varied diet, choosing from a wide range of different kinds of foods.
- Eat at least three pieces of fresh fruit a day, and two to three servings of fresh vegetables.
- Eat fast-fermenting and acid fruits on their own as snacks. Most soft fruits, including peaches, plums, mangoes, papayas, strawberries and melon, ferment quickly. High-acid fruits (although alkaline-forming) may also inhibit digestion of a carbohydrate; these include oranges, lemons, grapefruit and pineapple. All of these fruits require little digestion, releasing their natural fructose content quickly.
- Include a salad as a major part of one meal each day. Try to incorporate dark green leafy and root vegetables such as watercress, carrots, sweet potatoes, broccoli, Brussels sprouts, spinach, green beans or peppers, raw or lightly cooked.
- Eat plenty of the foods rich in antioxidants and phytochemicals, such as peas, broccoli, watercress, carrots and berries.
- Eat two servings daily of beans, lentils, tofu or 'seed' vegetables.
- Eat 80 per cent alkaline-forming foods, 20 per cent acid-forming foods (see page 7). This means eating large quantities of vegetables and fruit, and less concentrated protein foods such as beans, lentils and whole grains, meat, fish, cheese and eggs.

- Eat animal protein with vegetables. Concentrated protein such as meat, fish, hard cheese and eggs requires lots of stomach acid and a stay of about three hours in the stomach to be digested. So do not combine fast-releasing carbohydrates.
- Avoid refined carbohydrates, such as white sugar, white bread, bought cakes, biscuits etc.
- Choose free-range eggs and live yogurts. Keep dairy intake to a minimum.
- Eat as much raw food as possible. Raw organic fruits, vegetables, raw seeds, nuts and grains are particularly good for you.
- Choose seasonal produce that is fresh. Buy fresh foods in small quantities and buy them often, as keeping them destroys their nutrients.
- Choose organic fruit and vegetables. Be an opportunist and buy whatever looks good on the day. Do not worry about minor cosmetic blemishes, irregular sizing, minor bruises or the occasional insect. Store the food properly and eat it fresh. Organic food is now widely available, but for really fresh vegetables buy direct from a farm or through a box scheme.
- Eat organic meat and chicken; the animals are reared without the routine use of drugs, antibiotics and wormers which are commonly found in most conventional livestock farming.
- Drink at least 2 litres (3½ pints) of water a day. Add chunks of lemon, lime or orange to 'pep' it up, or freeze juices in ice cube trays and serve these in your water.
- Take frequent exercise and keep active.

Shopping and ingredients

Why buy organic?

A few years ago organic food could be found in very few outlets. Today all that has changed and organic foods can be bought everywhere, from major supermarkets and independent retailers to your local high street shops. Local box schemes and organic farm shops are popping up throughout the country and farmers' markets are beginning to appear in every town. In fact, it has never been easier to eat organic.

Organic food offers unparalleled benefits. When we buy organic we can be sure that the food is healthy and nutritious and that it has been produced in ways that sustain the environment, care for the animals and minimise pollution. We are reassured that organic food is natural food that we can trust.

I think one of the best reasons for buying organic foods is simply that it tastes so good. This is partly because organic produce is allowed to grow at its own pace, without chemical feeds or artificial nitrates (which increase the uptake of water). For example, organic carrots spend three times longer in the soil than conventional carrots, take up water at a slower rate and develop a higher fibre content, all of which contribute to extra flavour.

But undoubtedly there are also health reasons for eating organic. It has been proven in studies that organic produce contains fewer nitrates, minimal concentrations of pesticides and sometimes has higher levels of vitamin C, mineral and essential nutrients.

Many scientists believe that fruit and vegetables are only as good as the soil in which they are grown. Minerals pass from the soil to the plant and in turn help the plant to grow and produce vitamins. Non-organic farming methods rob the soil of nutrients and do not replace them. Phosphates found in fertilisers and pesticides bind to the minerals in the soil, making them less available to the plant. Also, if the land is used too frequently without periods of rest, the soil may become nutrient deficient. Farmers then turn to fertilisers, which will help plants to carry on growing, but without the full compliment of minerals. Consequently, the plants are not sufficiently full of vitamins and minerals and we can end up deficient too.

Organic foods contain the highest and best composition of minerals since the organic matter in the soil breaks down inorganic minerals (which your body cannot use) and turns them into an organic form (which it can). There is no way to compensate for the structural information missing when chemical farming has destroyed organic matter in soil. The components of plants – vitamins, minerals, essential fatty acids, carbohydrates, fibre and amino acids – have been bound together by nature to support one another. If this complex composition is destroyed it will undermine our own potential for energy, good looks and vitality.

A wide variety of pesticides are used in conventional agriculture, many of which can be extremely toxic to humans, promoting the onset of cancers and other life-threatening illnesses. These residues can occur in higher amounts in foods than allowed by government regulations. The cumulative effect of chemicals and toxic substances can be a huge strain on the kidneys and liver (our detoxifying organs) and can lead to the breakdown of various bodily systems. Organic food can help significantly to reduce the toxic load on our systems. This in turn will allow our bodies to spend less energy on digestion, leaving more energy for us to get on with our lives.

Organic farming is the only system to have totally rejected genetic engineering and GMO's are prohibited in any organic products.

Modern farming methods are changing. Animals are fed with processed foods, antibiotics and growth hormones before being slaughtered for human consumption. Pesticides, chemical fertilisers and factory farming have allowed a cocktail of toxic pollutants into the food chain. Chemically grown fruits, vegetables and cereals replete with toxic chemicals can deplete nutrients, disrupt enzyme reactions and pollute the body. A good deal of energy is wasted by the body in trying to disarm these alien and often toxic chemicals, some of which cannot be eliminated by our natural processes and start to accumulate in the body tissue.

Organic agriculture, on the other hand, is a safe, sustainable way of farming, producing healthy crops and livestock without causing damage to the environment. It avoids the use of artificial chemical fertilisers and pesticides on the land, instead relying heavily on developing a healthy, fertile soil and growing a mixture of crops. In this way the farm remains biologically balanced, with a wide variety of beneficial insects and other wildlife to act as natural predators for crop pests and a soil full of micro-organisms and earthworms. And organic animals are reared without the use of routine drugs, antibiotics and wormers, which are commonly found in most conventional livestock farming. Recent research also demonstrates that the widespread use of antibiotic growth promoters is a key factor behind the increasing incidence of drug-resistant disease in humans.

The quality of organic produce improves constantly; however, it does not necessarily match up to what people expect or have been used to. Likewise, flavours vary. Organic foods have their own characteristics. Fresh produce may not always be cosmetically perfect and though some organic foods taste similar to their conventional counterparts, others taste different because they *are* different. Because organic produce is closer to nature and grown in different ways from conventional food, its taste is influenced by a variety of factors including the season.

I believe that, as organic foods become the norm, it will be the organic versions that set the benchmarks for quality and flavour, and not the other way round. In the meantime, there is already plenty of choice and enough suppliers to please everyone and cater for all tastes; and in a rapidly growing market this means more and better choices for the foreseeable future.

Seasonal foods

To eat for energy we need to eat fresh whole foods that are as close to their natural state as possible. By choosing organic foods in season you are on the way to achieving this goal.

The following section includes a British food calendar, providing an indication of when a good variety of British ingredients are at their very best. There is so much British produce available, I have not listed everything, but hopefully this will give you a good guide as to the sorts of fresh produce to look out for each month. I am sure there are many of you who, like me, wish to bring back the seasons into our kitchens and benefit from our wonderful foods when they are at their best in terms of quality and value.

Freshness, good nutritional quality, great taste and value for money are just some of the benefits of buying British food in season. As we indulge in the delicacies that each new season has to offer, we are also helping to support the rural economy and ensure a living countryside for future generations to enjoy.

Some of you may be aware of the New Season for British Food campaign going on throughout Britain, organised by the National Farmer's Union (NFU). This campaign aims to encourage the public to rediscover the simple pleasure of eating locally produced food when it is in season. The New Season for British Food has been designed to feed the public's hunger for knowledge about seasons by encouraging shoppers to taste the best of each new season's food at events around the country, in farm shops, 'pick your own' outlets and farmers' markets.

All year availability for everything may be incredibly convenient but, in addition to question marks over quality and cost, much of the joy of cooking and eating is dampened by the lack of anything to look forward to. I get really excited about the simple pleasures of fresh ripe berries in summer mixed with thick creamy yogurt, the sweet crunch of an autumn apple, springtime-fresh asparagus or comforting roasted parsnips and potatoes. It is such a shame that these pleasures are dampened by the fact that the foods are available all year round in the shops rather than just during their seasons. Also, certain culinary traditions risk being forgotten when there is no arrival and no noticeable abundance of ingredients to celebrate.

I haven't mentioned organic chicken, as it seems to be in season most of the year without any noticeable variation in quality. The same applies to pork and beef, which I do not use very often in the recipes. Lamb is a different matter and I've noted the key times in the year when it's really good eating and should definitely be sought out. Don't fall for force-reared, so-called new season lamb at Easter; it's never seen grass and has only eaten pellets, so wait until the end of May.

I am not suggesting for one moment that imported ingredients should be pushed to one side, just that full advantage needs to be taken of home-grown foodstuffs when they are at their best. I am the first to admit that fruits such as mangoes and pineapples are both delicious and packed with vitamins. Indeed it is sometimes not only preferable to choose imported products over home-grown, but actually imperative, especially in the early months of the year when imported fruit really saves the day due to the scarcity of home-grown produce.

British Food Calendar

January

Fruit apples (dessert, cooking), citrus fruits, chestnuts, grapes, pears, rhubarb (forced)

Vegetables artichokes, beetroot, Brussels sprouts, cabbage and kale (all year round), carrots, celery, celeriac, chicory, horseradish (most of the year), kohlrabi, leeks, mushrooms (brown cap), onions (maincrop), parsnips, potatoes (maincrop), salsify, seakale, shallots, spring greens, swede, sweet potatoes (not British), turnips, yams (not British)

Herbs bay leaves, rosemary, sage, thyme (all of these herbs are grown throughout the year)

Fish cod, Dover sole, grey mullet, haddock, halibut, lemon sole, oysters, scallops, turbot

Poultry goose, guinea fowl (all year), turkey

Game wild duck, guinea fowl (all year), hare, partridge, pheasant, pigeon (all year), rabbit (all year), snipe, venison, wild boar (all year), quail (all year)

February

Fruit apples (dessert, cooking), chestnuts, citrus fruits, pears, rhubarb (forced)

Vegetables artichokes, beetroot, Brussels sprouts, cardoons, carrots, celery, celeriac, chard, chicory, curly kale, kohlrabi, leeks, mushrooms (brown cap), onions (maincrop), parsnips, potatoes (maincrop), salsify, seakale, shallots, spring greens, sweet potatoes (not British), swede, turnips, watercress, yams (not British)

Fish cod, Dover sole, grey mullet, haddock, halibut, oysters, brown shrimp, lemon sole, turbot

Meat lamb

Game wild duck, hare, partridge, pheasant, pigeon, rabbit, venison

Poultry goose

March

Fruit almonds, apples (dessert, cooking), chestnuts, citrus fruits, macadamias, pecans, rhubarb (forced)

Vegetables artichokes, beetroot, purple-sprouting broccoli, carrots, chicory, cucumbers, leeks, mushrooms (brown cap), onions (maincrop), parsnips, potatoes (maincrop), radishes, seakale, shallots, spring greens, swede, turnips, watercress

Herbs parsley

Fish halibut, mussels, oysters, wild salmon, scallops, brown shrimp, lemon sole, sea trout

Meat lamb

Game wild duck, hare

Poultry chicken

April

Fruit almonds, apples (cooking), chestnuts, gooseberries, lemons, loquats, macadamias, pecans, rhubarb (forced, outdoor), strawberries

Vegetables asparagus, purple-sprouting broccoli, carrots, cauliflower, cucumbers, leeks, mushrooms (brown cap), potatoes (maincrop), Jersey potatoes, radishes, seakale, sorrel, spinach, spring greens, watercress

Herbs basil, wild garlic, lovage, mint, mixed spice, rocket

Fish crab, halibut, lemon sole, spiny lobster (crawfish), mussels, edulis oyster, wild salmon, shrimps, brown trout, sea trout (salmon trout)

Meat lamb

Game gulls' eggs

May

Fruit almonds, apples (cooking), chestnuts, gooseberries, macadamias, pecans, raspberries, rhubarb (outdoor), strawberries

Vegetables asparagus, broccoli (sprouting), carrots (late spring onwards), cucumbers, Florence fennel, kohlrabi, mushrooms (brown cap), potatoes (maincrop), spring and welsh onions (mid-spring onwards), new potatoes, peas, radishes, rocket, sorrel, spinach, spring greens, spring onions, watercress

Herbs basil, chives, coriander, lemon balm, mint, parsley, tarragon

Fish crab, haddock, lobster, mussels, gigas oyster, prawns, salmon, brown shrimp, brown trout, sea trout

Meat lamb (new season)

Game duck

June

Fruit almonds, apples (cooking), cherries (look out for these at the end of May), chestnuts, currants elderflower, gooseberries, loganberries, macadamias, pecans, raspberries, rhubarb (outdoor), strawberries, tayberries

Vegetables asparagus, beetroot broad beans, Chinese cabbage, carrots (new season), celery, courgettes, cucumbers, Florence fennel, lettuce, peas, potatoes (new), radishes, rocket, salad leaves, sorrel, spinach, spring onions, turnips (new season, summer and autumn)

Fish bass, crab, Dover sole, grilse (young salmon), haddock, halibut, grey mullet, lobster, gigas oyster, prawns, salmon, brown shrimp, sea trout

Poultry duckling

Cheese goat's cheese

July

Fruit almonds, bilberries, blackberries, blackcurrants, blueberries, cherries, chestnuts, currants, gooseberries, loganberries, macadamias, mangoes (not British), peaches and nectarines, pecans, raspberries, redcurrants, rhubarb (outdoor), strawberries, tayberries, whitecurrants

Vegetables globe artichoke, beetroot (new season), broad beans, French beans, runner beans, broccoli, capsicums and chillies, Chinese cabbage, cucumber, Florence fennel, garlic (mid-summer onwards), peas, radishes, rocket, marsh samphire, sorrel, spinach, spring onions, tomatoes, turnips

Herbs basil, chervil, chives, coriander, dill, mint, parsley, tarragon

Fish sea bass, crab (spider), grisle, haddock, halibut, grey mullet, lobster, gigas oyster, prawns, salmon, brown shrimp, Dover sole, brown trout, turbot

Poultry duckling

August

Fruit almonds, apricots, bilberries, blackberries, blackcurrants, blueberries, cherries, chestnuts, currants, gooseberries, loganberries, macadamias, melons (not British), mulberries, peaches and nectarine, pecans, plums, raspberries, redcurrants, rhubarb (outdoor), strawberries, tayberries, whitecurrants

Vegetables artichokes, aubergines, broad beans, French beans, runner beans, beetroot, broccoli, capsicums and chillies, carrots, Chinese cabbage, cauliflower, celery, chard, courgettes, cucumber, Florence fennel, kohlrabi, leeks, lettuce, marrows, mushrooms (brown cap, wild), onions (pickling), peas, potatoes (new), pumpkin, radishes, rocket, shallots, sorrel, spinach, spring onions, squash, sweetcorn, tomatoes, turnips

Herbs basil, chervil, chives, coriander, dill, mint, parsley, tarragon, nasturtiums

Fish sea bass, crab, Dover sole, haddock, halibut, lobster, grey mullet, gigas oyster, prawns, salmon, brown shrimp, turbot

Game wild duck, quail, grouse, snipe

Poultry guinea fowl

Cheese Devon blue

September

Fruit almonds, apples (dessert, cooking), apricots, blackberries, blueberries, bullaces, cape gooseberries, crab apples, chestnuts, damsons, elderberries, figs, grapes, greengages, hazelnuts, macadamias, medlars, mulberries, peaches and nectarines, pears, pecans, plums, quinces, raspberries, rhubarb (outdoor), sloes, strawberries

Vegetables artichokes, aubergines, beetroot, broad beans, French beans, runner beans, broccoli, Chinese cabbage, capsicums and chillies, carrots, celery, chard, chicory, courgette, cucumber, kohlrabi, leeks, lettuce, marrow, mushrooms (brown cap, wild), onions, onions (pickling), potatoes (maincrop, new), pumpkin, radishes, rocket, shallots, sorrel, spinach, spring onions, squash, sweetcorn, swede, tomatoes, turnips, watercress

Herbs basil, chervil, chives, coriander, dill, mint, parsley, tarragon

Fish sea bass, cod, Dover sole, grey mullet, haddock, halibut, lobster, mussels, prawns, oysters, brown shrimp, turbot

Meat lamb

Game wild duck, grouse, hare, mallard, partridge, pigeon, rabbit, snipe

October

Fruit apples (dessert, cooking), blackberries, blueberries, bullaces, cape gooseberries, crab apples, damsons, elderberries, hazelnuts, figs, grapes, macadamias, medlars, mulberries, pears, pecans, quinces, raspberries, rowanberries, sloes, strawberries, walnuts

Vegetables aubergines, runner beans, beetroot, broccoli, capsicums and chillies, celeriac, chicory, chard, Chinese cabbage, corn salad, courgette, cucumber, kohlrabi, leeks, lettuce, marrow, mushrooms (brown cap, wild), onions (pickling, maincrop), parsnips, pak choi, sweet potatoes and yams (not British), potatoes (maincrop), pumpkin, radishes, rocket, shallots, spinach, squash, swede, sweetcorn, turnips, watercress

Herbs basil, chives, coriander, mint, parsley

Fish sea bass, cod, haddock, halibut, grey mullet, mussels, oysters, prawn, scallops, brown shrimp, Dover sole, turbot

Meat lamb

Game wild duck, geese, grouse, hare, partridge, pheasant, pigeon, rabbit, veal, venison

Poultry goose, guinea fowl

November

Fruit apples (dessert, cooking), brazil nuts, bullaces, cape gooseberries, chestnuts, damsons, filberts, figs, grapes, hazelnuts, macadamias, medlars, mulberries, pears, pecans, quinces, rhubarb (forced), sloes, walnuts

Vegetables Jerusalem artichokes, beetroot, broccoli, Brussels sprouts, Chinese cabbage, celeriac, chard, chicory, corn salad, courgette, kohlrabi, leeks, marrow, mushrooms (brown cap, wild), onions (pickling, maincrop), parsnips, potatoes, pumpkins, wood blewit mushrooms, shallots, spinach, squash, swede, turnips, watercress

Herbs basil, chives, coriander, mint, parsley

Fish sea bass, cod, Dover sole, grey mullet, haddock, halibut, mackerel, mussels, oysters, sprats, turbot

Game wild duck, hare, mallard, partridge, pheasant, pigeon, rabbit, snipe, woodcock, venison

Poultry goose, guinea fowl, turkey

December

Fruit apples (dessert, cooking), brazil nuts, cape gooseberries, citrus fruits, chestnuts, clementines, cranberries (not British), grapes, lychees (not British), macadamias, pears, quinces, rhubarb (forced), walnuts

Vegetables Jerusalem artichokes, beetroot, red cabbage, cardoons, celeriac, celery, chard, chicory, corn salad, curly kale, leeks, mushrooms (brown cap, wild), onions (maincrop), parsnips, sweet potatoes and yams (not British), potatoes, kohlrabi, salsify, Brussels sprouts, swede, white truffles, turnips

Herbs cinnamon

Fish sea bass, cod, Dover sole, grey mullet, haddock, halibut, lemon sole, mussels, oysters, scallops, turbot

Game deer, wild duck, hare, mallard, partridge, pheasant, pigeon, rabbit, snipe, venison, woodcock

Poultry goose, turkey

Cheese Stilton

I haven taken the seasons to be: spring – end March to June; summer – end June to end September; autumn – end September to beginning December; winter – December to end March

Ingredients

This list is a good selection of the ingredients used throughout the book. It is not intended to panic you into thinking you need to rush out and buy everything, but more to act as a guide to remind you of the ingredients that you may like to dabble with in the recipes.

Store cupboard

Seeds

Sesame, sunflower and pumpkin.

Nuts

Brazil, cashew, hazelnuts and almonds. Be sure that any nuts and seeds you buy are very fresh and unsalted (it is best to buy these in small quantities rather than keeping them for long periods of time). Store them in the refrigerator or freezer to protect their oils from oxidation. To really bring out their flavour, toast the nuts or seeds in a dry frying pan until golden, stirring or shaking the pan to prevent them from burning. Scatter over salads or just enjoy nibbling on them.

Nut spreads

Tahini (made from sesame seeds) and cashew nut butter contain protein, vitamins and minerals.

Seeds, grains and pulses for sprouting

Alfalfa, lentils (especially puy), mung or aduki beans and wheat. Buy a small bag of each and combine to make a flavourful sprout mix.

Seaweed

Seaweed contains minerals, protein and vitamins. Nori seaweed and konbu are both easy to use (make sushi, see page 105).

Standbys from a can

Sweetcorn (without added sugar), artichoke hearts, olives, capers, tuna fish (packed in water) and anchovies.

Coconut milk

It contains minerals and small quantities of B vitamins. Incidentally it is not the liquid inside a coconut, it is liquid pressed from grated coconut flesh and diluted with water, or obtained from dried coconut after it has been soaked in hot water, milk or a mixture of both.

Grains

Couscous, bulgar wheat and porridge oats. Couscous is a kind of hard wheat semolina that has been ground, then moistened and rolled in flour. Bulgar is a whole wheat that has been boiled until tender, then dried and ground. Both are excellent for quick lunches served with lots of fresh vegetables, salad ingredients and delicious dressings.

Beans and pulses

Chickpeas, cannellini beans, kidney beans, butter beans, broad beans, puy lentils and green lentils are my favourite (canned or dried). If you do use cans give the beans a good rinse under the tap to wash off the sugar or salt often found in their water.

Rice

Brown and basmati.

Pasta

Good for slow-released energy; choose a few favourites to keep in the cupboard.

Sauces

Mustards (whole grain), olive pastes, pesto, harissa, tamari (wheat-free soy sauce) and Rustica crushed tomatoes are, in my mind, essentials.

Swiss Vegetable Bouillon Powder

If you do not have time to make your own stock, this is the only alternative (stock cubes have a nasty artificial flavour in comparison).

Oils

Use olive oil for wok-frying foods. For your salad dressings use extra virgin olive oil ideally mixed fifty-fifty with pure cold-pressed flaxseed oil, an energy-enhancing addition. Flaxseed oil is the best polyunsaturated oil you can find for supplying essential fatty acids in your diet. You will need to ask in health food shops for it. It must be bought fresh and under refrigeration, then kept refrigerated once opened and used within weeks or it goes rancid. Fresh flaxseed oil taken either in capsules or mixed with extra virgin olive oil on your salads has been shown to clear up cases of premenstrual syndrome, asthma, allergies, water retention in women, skin conditions and also to enhance vitality – all within a month. But it doesn't work unless it is of the highest quality and absolutely fresh. Another favourite of mine for salad dressings is a good fresh walnut, hazelnut or sesame oil; just mix with a little lemon or lime juice. It is best to keep the nut oils refrigerated to stop them from going rancid.

Golden organic linseeds
Linseeds are an excellent source of essential fatty acids. Along with fibre complex they help free the intestinal wall of unwanted debris.

Vinegars
Rice wine, cider, champagne and balsamic. Champagne vinegar is available from supermarkets, but if you do have trouble finding it use white wine or rice wine vinegar instead. Balsamic requires spending a little extra cash in order to get a good dark, sweet, rich and deep flavour.

Spices
My advice is to keep small quantities of a selection of whole spices such as green cardamom pods, coriander seeds, black peppercorns, cinnamon sticks, nutmeg and dried chillies (see chillies in the fridge section) and grind them as and when required. Star anise, saffron and vanilla pods are also useful.

Sea salt flakes (Maldon)
They have such a wonderful taste that you will find yourself using less than normal salt. The salt commonly available from supermarkets has often been highly processed to remove trace minerals and to keep it from clumping.

Raw honey
This is rich in vitamins, minerals and enzymes.

Unrefined sugars
It is not advisable to eat large quantities of any sort of sugar, but when you do eat it, it should be the right sort. I am not the first to say it and I certainly will not be the last, unrefined sugars are the only sugars to use. Look out for Billingtons or own label sugars (but check on the label that it says unrefined, otherwise you may be buying a white sugar that has been coloured brown).

Dried fruits
Dates, figs, apricots and raisins. Eat them for energy as well as the iron they supply and their high potassium content. Dates are a good source of fibre, folic acid, fruit sugar, iron and potassium. Figs are great for beta-carotene, cancer-fighting phytochemicals, fibre, iron and potassium. Prunes contain beta-carotene, fibre, iron, niacin, potassium and vitamin B6.

Olives
Black Niçoise olives (small, strong flavoured olives imported from France) and Kalamata olives (Greek).

Wheat germ
Vitamin E present in wheat germ helps the circulation in the body and the folic acid is excellent for women trying to conceive and those who are pregnant.

Pickled ginger
Not the bright pink kind: the colour indicates the presence of a nasty die.

Wasabi
Japanese horseradish with a real attitude.

Wine
A few bottles of white and red wine.

Herb teas
Peppermint, ginger etc.

Fridge

Spring water
See Introduction for details about why we should drink water.

Live yogurt
Contains beneficial bacteria, calcium, protein, riboflavin and zinc. Choose yogurt made from goat's or sheep's milk. Cow's milk is much harder to digest and mucus forming.

Cottage cheese
Very easy and quick snack food that contains B vitamins, calcium, folic acid, magnesium, protein and vitamin A.

Houmous
Chickpeas are rich in fibre, iron and magnesium.

Soya milk or organic milk
There are lots of different brands of soya milk available; I really advise you to taste a variety.

Tofu
Tofu can make a good base for dips or creamy dressings.

Mixed salad leaves
Keep a bag of mixed leaves or a selection of lettuce. They can add bulk to salads while providing calcium, folic acid, phosphorous, potassium and vitamins A and C. Watercress contains anti-bacterial mustard oils, beta-carotene, iron, vitamins C and E.

Celery
Has a calming effect, helping to eliminate stress and keep blood pressure low. It also contains potassium and vitamin C.

Alfalfa sprouts
Keep a pack in the fridge for throwing over salads. They are useful things that contain calcium, vitamins A, C, E, B complex and K.

Spices

Fresh ginger
One of the most versatile and valuable of spices. The ancient Greeks used it for digestive problems and as an antidote to poisoning, while medieval herbalists valued its warming properties highly. In ancient Chinese medicine and the traditional Ayurvedic healing of India it is a vital ingredient. This knobbly root keeps best if wrapped in kitchen paper and kept in a paper bag. When you choose fresh root ginger, make sure that it is firm to touch.

Garlic
The natural substances in garlic help to lower cholesterol and are also antibacterial and anti-fungal. They have also been seen to ward off chest infections.

Chillies
The capsaicin in the chilli is a remarkable circulatory stimulant. It has a dramatic effect on blood flow.

For a general guide to the heat of chillies; skinny and thin chillies are hotter than those with broad shoulders, although the scotch bonnet proves otherwise. Make sure you taste the food as you are making it and add a little – you can always add more. As soon as you add an ingredient like coconut milk or any other high-fat liquid to chilli or chilli paste the taste will become milder.

Another interesting fact about chillies is that fresh chillies with wrinkled skins are hotter than the smooth kind. But if dried chillies are wrinkled they are often sweeter than the smooth hotter ones.

Lemon grass
Just remember to bash the thin end before using as this helps to release its citrus flavour.

Horseradish
Contains a powerful natural substance, sinigrin, which is an antibiotic that helps to protect against infections.

Saffron
I love this pretty spice and the wonderful colour it washes all over foods. It contains volatile constituents that help soothe menstrual cramps and pain.

Vegetable rack

I am not suggesting that you rush out and buy all of these, just keep an eye out for them and buy a selection as and when you see them.

Kale
Contains beta-carotene, calcium, cancer-fighting phytochemicals, vitamin C, folic acid, iron and phosphorous.

Spinach
Contains beta-carotene, cancer-fighting phytochemicals, carotenoids, iron and folic acid.

Beetroot
The red colour in beetroot is similar to that of haemoglobin in blood and is a traditional effective treatment for anaemia, leukaemia and cancer in Eastern Europe.

Beet tops are iron-rich. The massive potassium content of beetroot with its leaves helps keep blood pressure low, vital for a long and active life. Contains beta-carotene, calcium, folic acid, magnesium, potassium and vitamin A.

Radishes
The sulphur content in radishes is anti-bacterial and their bitter flavour stimulates the flow of saliva, crucial to the prevention of gum disease. Radishes also stimulate the gall bladder to increase the release of bile, as well as stimulating the liver. They are specifically healing to the mucous membranes of the nose, sinuses and throat, while protecting against chest infections.

Asparagus
Contains substantially large amounts of protein for a vegetable: as much, in fact, as the same weight of rice or corn on the cob. It is therefore an excellent slow-release energy and has the added benefit of being a diuretic with cleansing properties. As well as folic acid, it contains potassium, vitamin C and phosphorous.

Carrots
Cleanse the skin from the inside outwards and the fibre helps to stimulate the normal contractions of the large bowel, hastening elimination. The complex carbohydrates in the carrots break down slowly, providing a gradual release of energy.

Cabbages
Contains cancer-fighting phytochemicals, folic acid, potassium, vitamins A, C and E.

Fennel and chicory
Have an influence on the liver and kidney functions – they are perfect for easing bloating that often accompanies periods. It is the volatile oils in fennel that give it its unique flavour as well as diuretic, cleansing and digestive properties.

Leeks
Sulphur compounds in leeks help reduce cholesterol and improve blood flow. The phytochemicals in the leek stimulate good digestion and improve nutrient absorption to increase energy levels.

Tomatoes
Good source of beta-carotene, lycopene, potassium, vitamins C and E.

Sweet potato
Contains beta-carotene and other carotenoids, cancer-fighting phytochemicals, protein, vitamins C and E.

Fruit bowl

Once again, it is not necessary to rush out to the local market or shops to stock up on all of the following fruits. Take a look at some of the benefits of each and then choose recipes to help you start to easily incorporate them into the diet. Each fruit has its own specific health-benefiting properties and they are all needed in one way or another when we are eating for energy and a healthy lifestyle.

Apples
Pectin in apples helps remove impurities from the system and they are rich in vitamins and minerals, including vitamin C and potassium.

Apricots
Good source of beta-carotene as well as iron, potassium and soluble fibre.

Pears
The dark green thicker-skinned pears contain more fibre and pectin, the golden yellow Williams version is sweeter with more sugar. As well as soluble fibre they are a great source of vitamin C.

Strawberries
Contain anti-arthritic phytochemicals, beta-carotene and vitamins C and D.

Grapes
Very effective cleansers for the skin, liver, intestines and kidneys, due to their potent properties which counter excessive mucus in your system. Easily digested and a quick source of energy and rich in minerals.

Pineapple
Contains a high concentration of bromelin, an enzyme that supports the action of hydrochloric acid in the stomach and helps to break down protein wastes in the system. Eating pineapple is also believed to soothe internal inflammation, accelerate tissue repair, regulate the glandular system, clear mucus and aid digestion.

Papaya and mango
Papaya and mango are good for cleansing the alimentary canal and helping digestive disorders. They, like other tropical fruits such as mangosteen, passion fruit and guava, supply us with antioxidants.

Peaches
Contain beta-carotene, flavonoids, potassium and vitamin C.

Watermelon
A wonderful diuretic and great for washing your system clean.

Cantaloupe and Ogen melons
Contain folic acid, potassium, small amounts of B vitamins, vitamins A and C.

Oranges
They also contain potassium, thiamine, vitamin B6 and C.

Passion fruit
Contains beta-carotene, vitamin C and phytochemicals.

Kiwi fruit
Contains huge amounts of carotenoids which are protective and energy-enhancing, beta-carotene, fibre, potassium and vitamin C.

Plums
Contain beta-carotene, malic acid (an effective aid to digestion), vitamins C and E.

Bananas
One of the fruits that contains chromium, a mineral essential for energy metabolism. Good source of energy, fibre, folic acid, magnesium, potassium and vitamins B6 and C.

Blackcurrants
Anti-inflammatory and cancer-fighting phytochemicals, carotenoids and vitamin C.

Blueberries
Contain vitamin C and carotenoids.

Cranberries
Contain cancer-fighting phytochemicals, specific urinary anti-bacterial and vitamin C.

Cherries
Contain cancer-fighting phytochemicals, flavonoids, magnesium, potassium and vitamin C.

Grapefruit
Good source of beta-carotene and vitamin C.

Fresh lemons and limes
Choose ones that feel heavy for their size, are fragrant and have a close-grained peel. If you are using the zest (the yellow part of the peel) try to buy organic lemons.

Fresh herbs

If you can grow your own herbs, do. My advice is to sow your own seeds rather than trying to keep small pots alive.

Fresh mint and parsley
Both have a healing effect on the entire digestive system and are calming to the central nervous system.

Parsley
This has legendary diuretic powers to stimulate the kidney and eliminate toxins.

Chives
Contain antiseptic and antifungal sulphur compounds, beta-carotene and vitamin C.

Coriander
Contains cleansing aromatic oils and digestive promoting constituents, also anti bacterial properties.

Sage
Stimulates liver function and is a powerful antiseptic due to its high content of an essential oil.

Rosemary
Improves memory and concentration.

Thyme
Good antiseptic.

Basil
Like so many of the herbs, basil has an ancient history as a medicine and it energises both mind and body (see pesto recipe on page 85).

Freezer

I could go on and on here: I love my freezer and I can always dip into it and find something that can be turned into supper. The obvious foods to store in a freezer are fresh fruits and vegetables; buy extra when they are in season and freeze until needed. Also, if you have time to make your own bread, it freezes really well and it is always such a treat to eat fresh bread from the oven.

Frozen berries
Whizz in a food processor with soya ice cream or crush and mix with a sorbet and serve in wine glasses for a fruity sensation.

Part-baked loaf of bread
Whoever pops in unexpectedly will be more than happy when they smell fresh bread baking. They will be even more delighted to taste fresh, squidgy bread drizzled with olive oil and a little garlic, served with some fresh soup.

Sorbets and ice creams
There are many good fruit sorbets to choose from. Look for the ones that have a high fruit content and check on the label for animal free additives. My favourite ice cream is soyice made from soya instead of dairy ingredients.

Young broad beans or petit pois
If you don't have time to go to the green grocer on your way home, you will at least have something sweet and green on your plate for your supper.

Frozen puff and filo pastry
There is no need to make these pastries from scratch, they take far too long.

1 Breakfasts and drinks

Breakfasts and drinks

Eating a good breakfast is important for energy; it also helps to wake up the brain. If you work without eating a small breakfast you may turn to artificial stimulants such as coffee, chocolate or sugar. It is a good idea to eat some form of complex carbohydrate for breakfast as these provide a steady stream of energy in the form of glucose throughout the morning.

We may not have long in the morning to make or eat breakfast, but time is not always necessary. This section of recipes includes fresh fruit juices, fruit based recipes and recipes that are easy to prepare and which will literally feed your brain. Eating breakfast has been proven to improve memory, learning and even creativity.

Fresh fruit is excellent for breakfast food because:

- Fruit is high in vitamins, minerals and enzymes, and detoxifies our systems at a rapid rate. The morning is the best time for our bodies to naturally detoxify themselves, because the liver is most efficient between midnight and midday.
- Fruit maintains energy levels, because little energy is used to digest them. If you feel hungry and need more than just fruit, eat fruit and then leave at least thirty minutes before eating one of the carbohydrate or protein recipes.
- Fruit is a good source of potassium, which needs to be balanced with sodium for perfect health. Many people eat far too much sodium in the form of table salt. Eating good quantities of fruit can help to rebalance a body, improve its functions and make you feel more energetic.
- Your body can make good use of the natural combination of sugars and fibre in fruit without experiencing the blood sugar problems that can lead to fatigue.
- Fruit contains antioxidant vitamins (see Introduction) that help to fight against diseases such as cancer and heart disease.

Juices and smoothies

Fresh juices have not only been credited with fighting disease, but also with giving relief for headaches, fatigue, acne, bruising, tooth decay and anxiety. You do not need a juicer to make the following recipes; they can all be whizzed successfully in a blender or food processor. This makes life easier, and it means that you drink both the liquid and the fibre. If you do juice the fruit in a juicer, remember to eat the whole fruit as well for its fibre.

Juices can be absorbed within fifteen to twenty minutes of drinking them, so they are great for an energy boost at the start of the day. If you are out and about and fancy a juice from one of the juice bars, try to choose the real juice-packed variety, and occasionally those with frozen yogurt or ice cream.

The recipes

Mix and match these recipes according to the foods in season and your own personal tastes. For carbohydrates, choose muesli, granola and porridge recipes. For protein, see if the omelette, scrambled eggs or other dishes like kippers with parsley and pepper tickle your fancy. I have included a few ideas for fruit purées and sundaes that include yogurt, because yogurt helps to keep the correct balance of intestinal flora in the gut. Yogurt is easier for us to digest than milk, partly because the milk protein in yogurt has been partially broken down by the bacteria. Try to choose yogurts made from soya, sheep's milk or goat's milk. Cow's milk is harder to digest and more mucus forming.

Drinks

For juices to deliver their greatest possible benefits use the freshest products available and enjoy!

Top tips:

Drink water as soon as you wake up so that you can achieve the goal of drinking 2 litres (3½ pints) of water before the end of the day.

Citrus juices help to remove some of the unwanted bacteria from the digestive tract and encourage the growth of beneficial bacteria.

Fast fermenting fruit include berries, cherries, mangoes, papaya, peaches, pears and strawberries. Slow fermenting fruit include apples, bananas and coconut.

Always dilute fruit juices with natural spring water for children – their digestive system is not as strong.

Mango and coconut smoothie

Coconut and mango is a delicious combination and the lime cuts through the flavour so that it is not too sweet. The beauty with this smoothie is that it travels really well, so you can make it and take to work or the pitch for half time.

Serves: 4
Preparation time: 10 minutes

2 large ripe mangoes
1 x 400 ml can coconut milk
juice of 1 lime
crushed ice

Cut the mangoes in half widthways, twist and pull apart – the stone will be left in one side. Cut around the stone to release the flesh and pull it out (in much the same way as you would stone a peach). Scoop out the flesh, put into a food processor, add the coconut milk and lime juice and whizz until smooth and frothy. Serve on lots of crushed ice.

Pineapple, grapefruit and passion fruit smoothie

Both of these smoothie recipes are suitable for people with dairy allergies. This fruity number is packed with vitamins. If you really don't like the look of passion fruit pips, sieve the juice from the fruit and throw away the seeds.

Serves: 4
Preparation time: 10 minutes

550 g/1¼ lb fresh pineapple
600 ml/1 pint freshly squeezed grapefruit juice
6 passion fruit

Peel the pineapple and cut the flesh into pieces. Whizz the pineapple in a blender or processor until smooth, add the grapefruit juice, mix together and pour into a jug. Cut the passion fruit in half, scoop the juice and pips into the pineapple mixture, mix together and serve.

Top tip:

Pineapples are good at aiding digestion because of the enzyme bromelain. You get approximately 150 ml/5 fl oz of pineapple juice from 450 g/1 lb of pineapple fruit.

Kiwi, banana and strawberry smoothie

Bart's spices make a coconut milk that is 88 per cent fat free. Look out for the fresh British strawberries during June, July and August when they are at their maximum tastiness, and enjoy a big bowl of them for breakfast or a quick snack.

Serves: 2
Preparation time: 10 minutes

1 kiwi
100 g/3½ oz strawberries, hulled and roughly chopped
2 small ripe bananas, peeled and sliced
200 ml/7 fl oz low fat coconut milk
50 ml/2 fl oz low fat yogurt (optional)
juice of 1 lime

Cut the kiwi in half, then scoop the flesh into a food processor or blender. Add the other ingredients and whizz until smooth.

Papaya, peach and passion fruit smoothie

This is low fat, cleansing and very good for the digestion. Check your papaya is ripe by the aroma – it should smell of the fruit and if you press it gently, the fruit should give slightly if it is ripe.

Serves: 2
Preparation time: 10 minutes

1 papaya
1 peach
2 passion fruit
150 ml/5 fl oz freshly squeezed orange juice

Peel the papaya, remove the seeds and put the flesh into a blender. Wash the peach, halve, remove the stone, chop the flesh and add to the blender. Halve the passion fruit and scoop the seeds straight into the blender with the orange juice. Blend until smooth. Serve poured over ice cubes with the remaining passion fruit over the top, and a stirrer.

Top tip:

I love papaya for many reasons: it contains several enzymes, principally papain, which helps with the digestion of proteins; it is also a real energy booster, a good cleanser for the internal organs and it helps to revive the appetite. I discovered just how effective this fruit is on my honeymoon when my husband and I were both affected by the water and food in Zanzibar, he in one way and me in the exact opposite. Towards the end of the holiday, we visited a woman at the hotel who specialised in alternative health – I was prescribed to take papaya flesh and the seeds and David just the fruit. Needless to say, this one fruit completely sorted us out.

Pineapple and coconut milk

The texture of this drink is quite thick so you may wish to add a little milk. It is delicious with cereal.

Serves: 2
Preparation time: 5 minutes

½ medium pineapple
30 g/1½ oz fresh coconut (or creamed)
150 ml/5 fl oz organic low fat natural yogurt
honey, to taste (optional)

Peel the pineapple, reserving a thin slice for the top. Chop the rest of the fruit and put into a food processor with the coconut. Blend, add the yogurt and blend again for a few seconds. Pour into a glass and serve. Add a little honey if you feel that it needs to be sweeter.

Cranberry and orange

Watch out for fruit juices that are loaded with sugar; wherever possible make your own juices using fresh fruit.

Serves: 2
Preparation time: 5 minutes

2 oranges
125 g/4 oz fresh cranberries
1 tsp clear honey

Use a sharp knife to cut the bottom and top off the oranges, then peel the skin and white pith away from the fruit, working your way around the fruit. Cut the oranges into chunks and put into a food processor, add the cranberries and honey and blend until smooth. Serve over ice.

Top tip:

Cranberries are a natural diuretic and urinary tract cleanser; they increase the urine's acidity, helping to destroy bacteria.

Melon madness

This looks amazing and will kick-start you into any day.

Serves: 2
Preparation time: 10 minutes

300g/11 oz watermelon chunks
½ cantaloupe melon, peeled and seeded, flesh cut into chunks
1 beetroot, peeled and cut into chunks

Put all the ingredients in a food processor and whizz until smooth. Pour into tall glasses and serve.

Top tip:

Melons are excellent cleansers for the bladder and kidneys.

Melon with ginger

This is really light and refreshing. Ginger is a fabulous root that helps to cleanse the system, especially at the beginning of the day.

Serves: 2
Preparation time: 5 minutes

½ canteloupe melon, peeled
2.5 cm/1 inch fresh root ginger, peeled and finely chopped
juice of ½ lime
sparkling spring water

Put the melon, ginger and lime juice into a food processor or blender and whizz until smooth. Add enough spring water to reach the desired consistency.

Orange berry blast

This is very easy and quick and only needs two fruits. The combination of orange and strawberry is a marriage made in heaven.

Serves: 1
Preparation time: 5 minutes

1 orange, peeled
150 g/5 oz strawberries, hulled

Using a sharp knife, cut the tops and bottoms off the orange. Then cut the skin away from the fruit and segment, leaving the white pith behind. Put the two fruits into a food processor or blender and whizz until smooth.

Let's go nutty

Serves: 1
Preparation time: 5 minutes

50 g/2 oz almonds, husks removed
150 ml/5 fl oz water
3 dates, stoned
3 figs
drop vanilla extract
honey, to taste

Put the almonds and water into a food processor and whizz until smooth. Add the rest of the ingredients and whizz again. Sweeten to taste with honey.

Paradise punch

Guaranteed to whisk you off to the Caribbean – just let your imagination run riot.

Serves: 2
Preparation time: 5 minutes

½ mango
½ banana, peeled
300g/11 oz pineapple
175ml/6 fl oz ice water, white grape juice, or another variety of juice

Cut the mango in half widthways, twist and break apart, then remove the stone. Scoop the flesh into a food processor or blender. Slice the banana and add to the mango. Peel the pineapple and slice the flesh into pieces, add to the fruit and whizz until smooth. Add enough water or juice until it is the right consistency.

Kiwi mania

There are so many delicious combinations that you can make with fresh fruit.

Serves: 2
Preparation time: 5 minutes

2 ripe kiwi fruit
450 g/1 lb honeydew melon
175 ml/6 fl oz water
4 sprigs mint

Peel the kiwi fruit and put the flesh straight into a food processor or blender. Cut the honeydew melon in half, scoop out the seeds and add the flesh to the kiwi fruit. Add a little spring water and whizz until smooth. Add enough spring water to reach your desired consistency, pour into glasses and drop in fresh sprigs of mint.

Papaya with passion fruit and lime

This is a quick way to get some fresh papaya into your system. Lime juice really brings out the flavour of papaya.

Serves: 2
Preparation time: 5 minutes

2 papayas
juice of ½ lime
2 passion fruit
sparkling or still spring water

Cut the papaya in half, scoop out the seeds and put the flesh into a food processor or blender. Add the lime juice and passion fruit juice and mix until blended. Add enough water to taste.

Carrot-apple zinger

Carrot juice stimulates the digestion and is a great tonic and rejuvenator.

Serves: 2
Preparation time: 5–10 minutes

4 carrots
2 apples, cored and cut into chunks
5 cm/2 inch piece fresh root ginger, peeled
still spring water

Trim the carrots and peel. Cut the carrots into chunks and put into a food processor or blender. Add the apples and ginger, whizz until smooth. Add enough water to taste and serve.

Top tip:

Carrots, as their colour suggests, have an excellent source of vitamin A (beta-carotene).

Fruit smoothies

Berry soup

Blueberry buttermilk pancakes

Nutty fruity slice

Green juice

When you are choosing spinach or other greens, make sure that the leaves look a fresh, dark green colour with no sign of wilting.

Serves: 2
Preparation time: 10 minutes

500 g/1¼ lb fresh greens such as spinach, kale or chard
1 cucumber, peeled and cut up
1 apple, cored and cut up
100 g/3½ oz parsley sprigs
200 g/7 oz green cabbage, shredded
sea salt flakes, freshly ground black pepper (optional)

Tear the fresh greens into a food processor, add the other ingredients and whizz to a juice. You may like to season with sea salt flakes and freshly ground black pepper.

Top tip:

Spinach is a great source of vitamin A and folic acid. The chlorophyll in green plants is good for the blood, a good cleanser and a mild laxative.

Spicy vegetable juice cocktail

Wherever possible, sneak beetroot into your diet – it is a fabulous cleanser and tonic.

Serves: 4
Preparation time: 5 minutes

2 large ripe tomatoes
2 celery stalks, trimmed
1 sweet red pepper, cored and seeded
2 carrots, trimmed
1 cucumber
1 beetroot, trimmed
1 bunch radishes, trimmed
1 jalapeno pepper, seeded and finely chopped
1 lemon, cut into chunks, to serve

Cut all of the vegetables into small pieces and put into a food processor or blender. Whizz until smooth, squeeze in lemon juice to taste and serve with wedges of lemon.

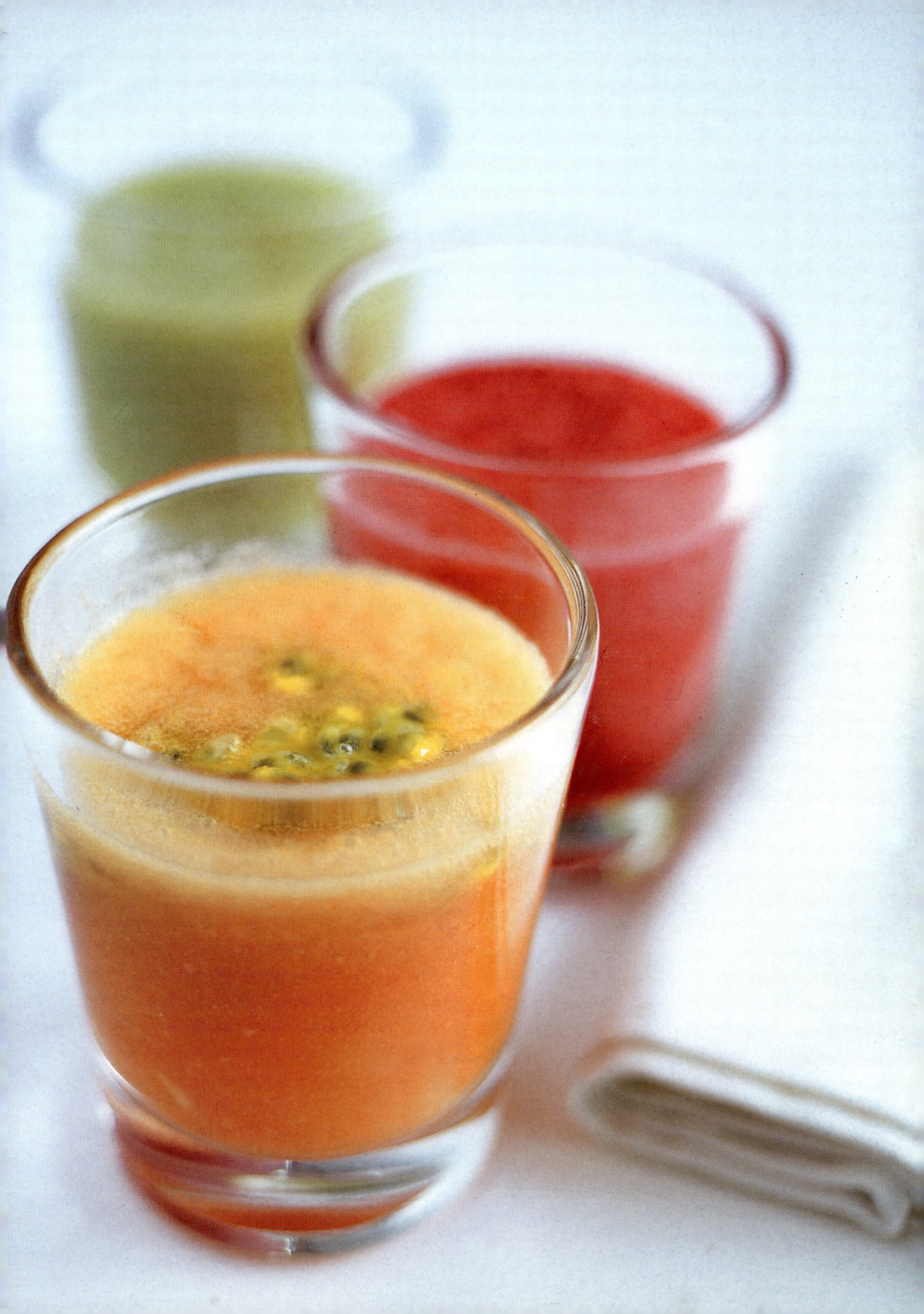

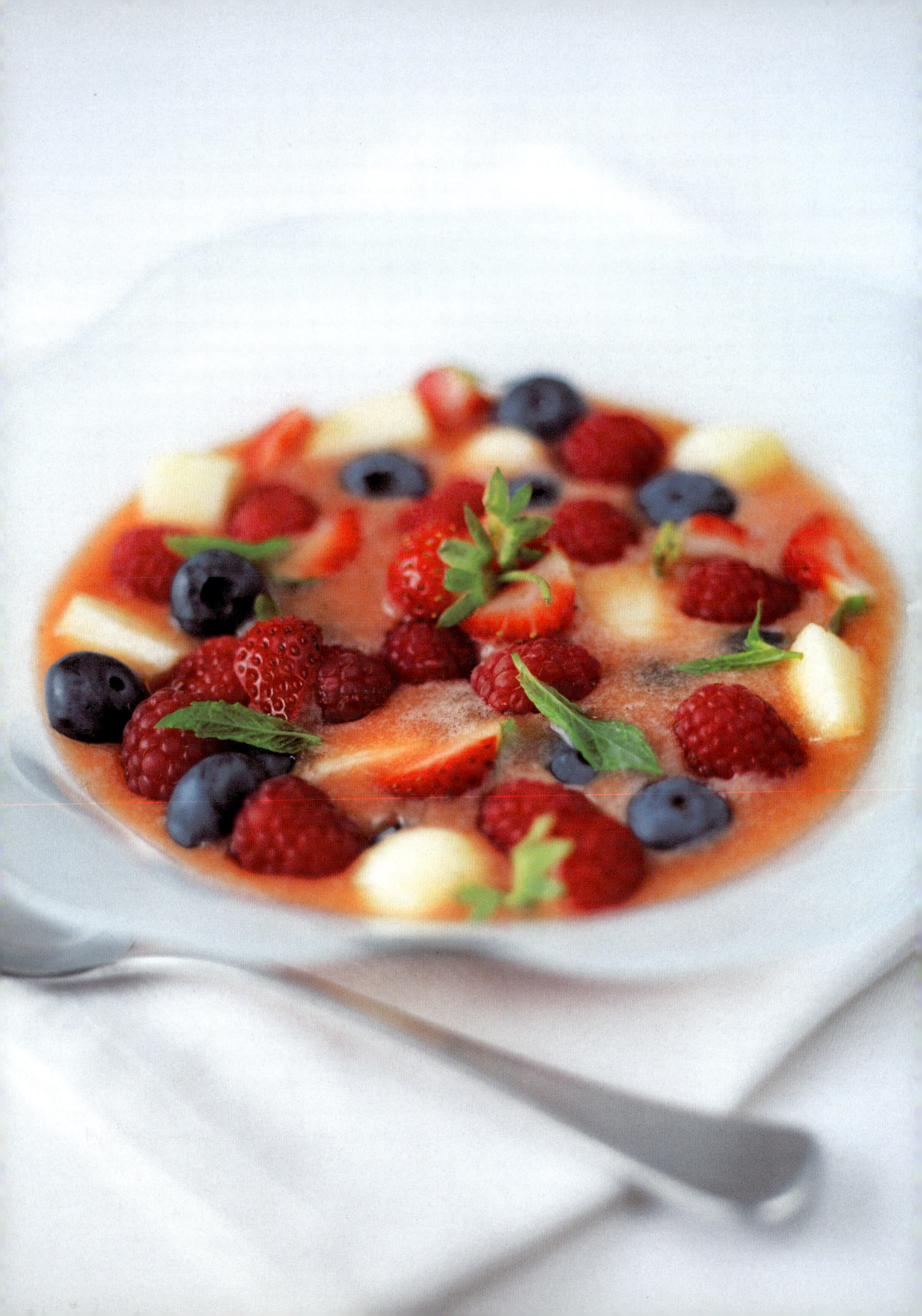

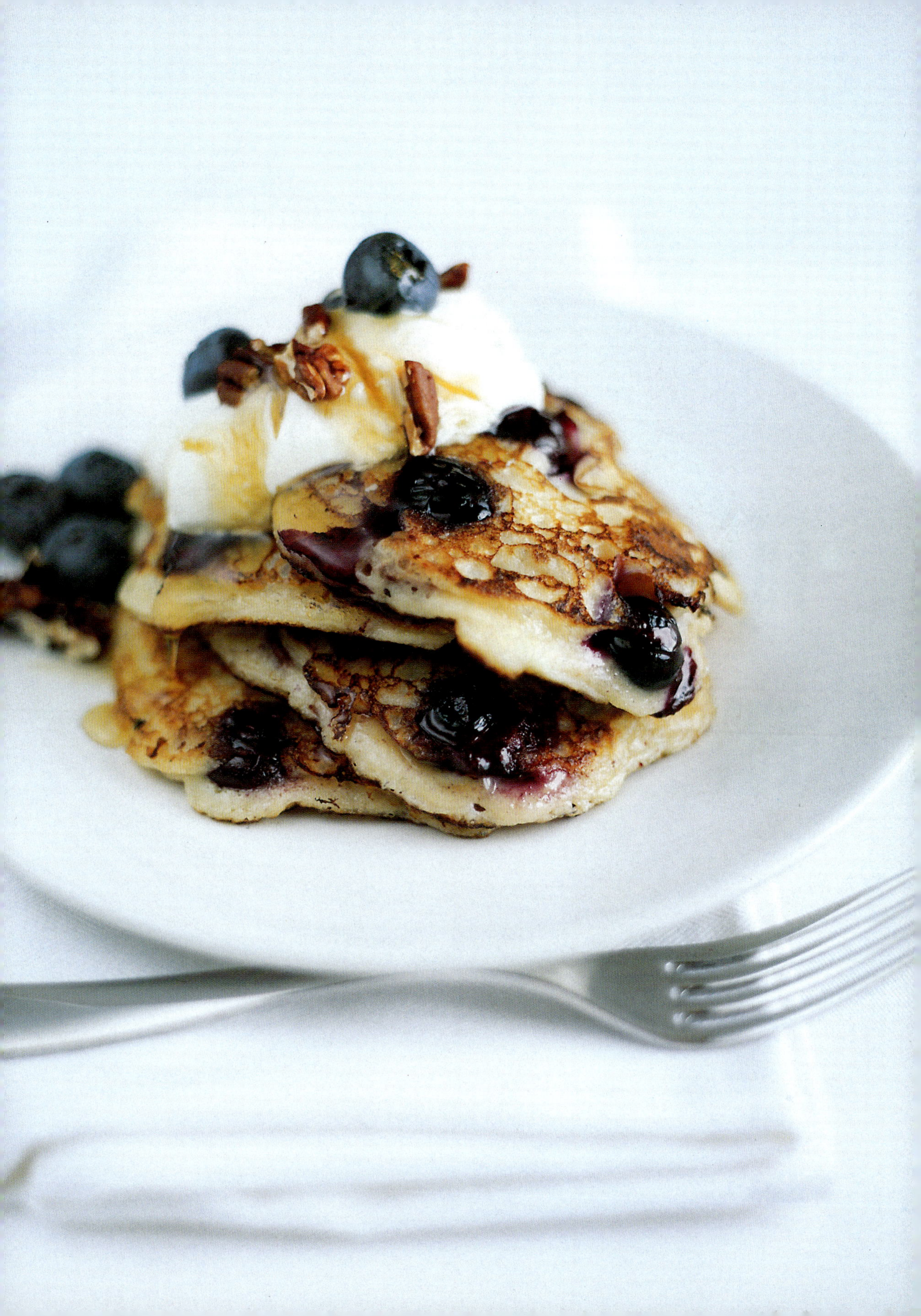

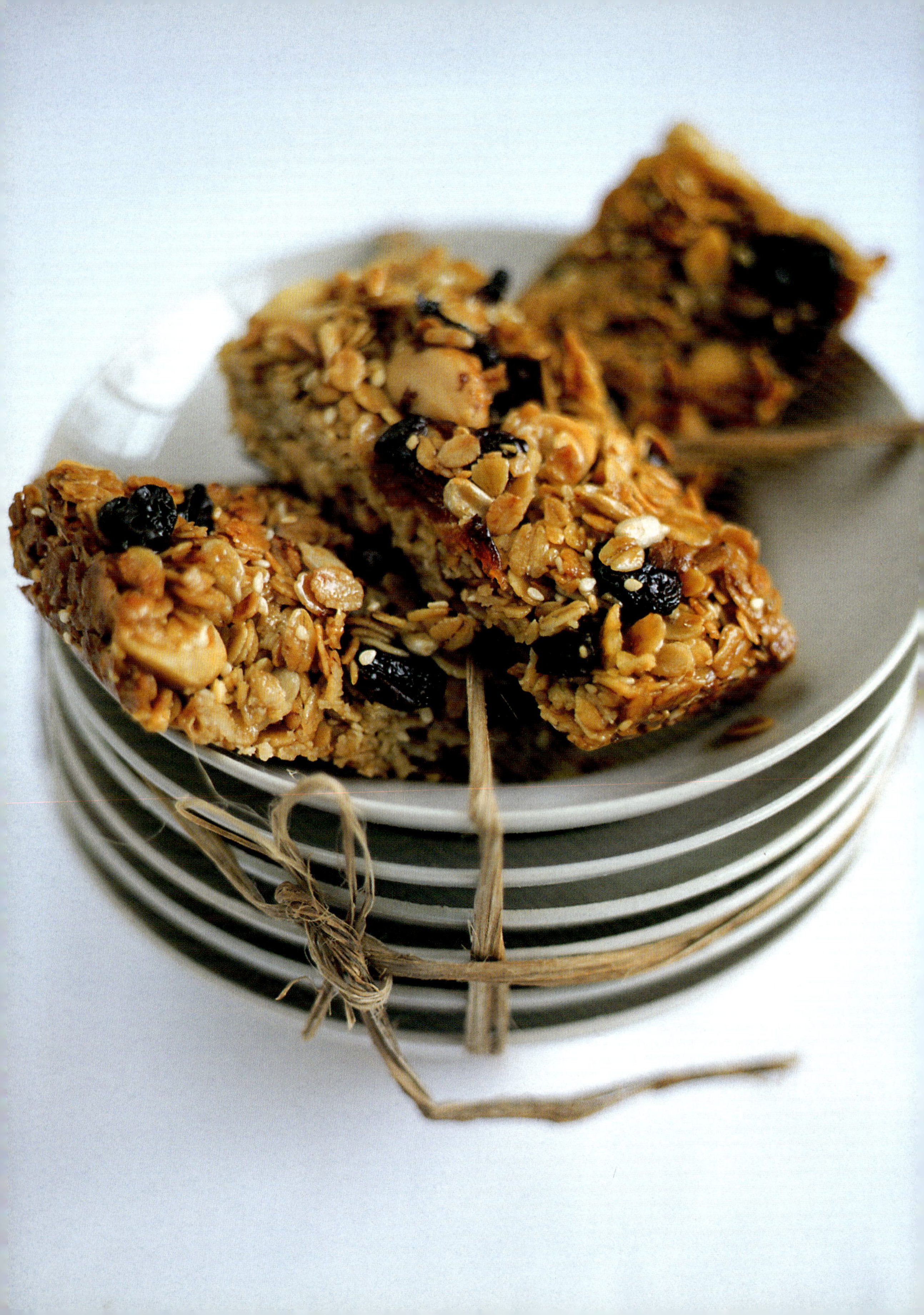

Quick and fruity dishes

Spiced apple sauce

This dish is low in calories and fat. It makes a perfect breakfast served with yogurt and/or a sprinkling of granola. Alternatively, spoon on to a bowl of porridge.

Serves: 4
Preparation time: 10 minutes
Cooking time: 15 minutes

8 Cox's or Bramley apples, peeled, cored and cut into chunks
150 ml/5 fl oz apple juice
1 tsp fresh minced ginger
1½ tsp cinnamon
½ tsp allspice
½ tsp cloves
1 star anise
lemon juice, to taste

Put everything into a large heavy-based saucepan. Heat gently over a medium heat until apples are tender, approximately 15 minutes, stirring occasionally. Remove the star anise and mash to the texture you desire with a potato masher. This is delicious with yogurt, porridge or granola.

Top tip:

Apples are excellent for detoxifying the body and helping to remove impurities from the system. They are also good for strengthening the liver and digestive system and for stimulating body secretions.

Rhubarb compôte

Rhubarb marries really well with both orange and ginger. There are two types of rhubarb, from the culinary viewpoint – forced and garden. Forced rhubarb appears in January and is sold throughout the spring. Garden rhubarb starts to appear in April and is normally available until the end of June.

Serves: 4
Preparation time: 15 minutes
Cooking time: 10–15 minutes

450 g/1 lb rhubarb
juice of 1 large orange
1 vanilla bean, split
sprinkling of soft brown sugar, to taste

Chop the rhubarb into chunks and put into a saucepan. Pour over the orange juice, add the split vanilla bean and then add sugar to taste. Cover and simmer gently for 10–15 minutes, or until cooked, but still holding its shape.

Top tip:

Be careful not to overcook the fruit: it will go mushy if is left in the pan for too long. This recipe is written to serve four people, however if you have more than 450 g/1 lb of rhubarb, cook it all at the same time. Leave to cool and then freeze in small portions. Serve with yogurts and/or granola.

Oranges with lavender

Lavender is becoming more popular as a culinary herb; it adds a very subtle sweet perfume and flavour to the fruit.

Serves: 4
Preparation time: 20 minutes (plus chilling time)

4 large oranges
4 blood oranges or mineolas
1 lemon
1 tbsp dried lavender, picked through for any bits

Cut the tops and bottoms off the oranges. Peel the oranges with a sharp serrated knife following the curve of the fruit, making sure you remove all of the bitter white pith. Slice the fruit into circles or chunks as you prefer, removing any pips as you go. Put the fruit into a bowl and pour over the juice of the lemon. Sprinkle over the lavender and then mix well, but gently. Refrigerate for a couple of hours before serving. Allow the dish to come to room temperature before eating.

Top tip:

You only need a little lavender to add flavour, too much and it can ruin a dish by making it astringent. Ideally, use your own lavender from a plant that you know has not been sprayed with pesticides or subjected to heavy pollution. Alternatively, buy lavender form a herbalist who knows that it is to be used in cooking.

Berry soup

This could be a breakfast, light lunch or starter. If you want to serve it as a dessert, add scoops of sorbet or ice cream to the middle and, for a real flourish, pour sparkling wine over the top. Watch the guests' faces as the sorbet bubbles and fizzes.

Serves: 4
Preparation time: 15 minutes
Cooking time: 15 minutes

200 ml/7 fl oz fresh pineapple juice
100 ml/3½ fl oz smoothie (buy a good smoothie or make your own using a handful of fresh strawberries, juice of 1 orange and a banana, whizzed in a food processor until smooth)
100 ml/3½ fl oz freshly squeezed orange juice
2 apples, peeled, cored and chopped into bite-sized pieces
1 star anise pod
juice of ½ lime
350 g/12 oz assorted berries (raspberries, blueberries, strawberries)
handful small fresh mint leaves, roughly torn

Put the pineapple juice, smoothie, orange juice, apple and star anise in a saucepan. Bring to the boil and gently simmer for about 5–10 minutes or until the apple is firm but tender. Transfer to a large bowl to cool. Remove the star anise pod. Stir through the lime juice, berries and mint leaves.

Top tip:

Star anise is a star shaped spice with an aniseed flavour. It is often used in Chinese cookery.

Hot fruit compôte with vanilla yogurt

I have made this compôte on numerous occasions for friends and it has been a winner every time. The fruit starts to caramelise and go all soft and gooey with a delicious flavour of wine in each bite. Serve the fruit in tall glasses, spoon the thick creamy yogurt on top and dust with a little cinnamon. It is so delicious you could serve this as a dessert instead of breakfast.

Serves: 4
Preparation time: 20 minutes
Cooking time: 40 minutes

350 g/12 oz dried apricots
300 ml/10 fl oz red wine
250 ml/8 fl oz water
500 ml/17 fl oz apple juice
5 cloves
½ tsp nutmeg
1 cinnamon stick
3 tbsp runny honey
2 large oranges
1 lemon
4 tbsp thick Greek yogurt (with a drop vanilla extract, optional)
large pinch ground cinnamon, to serve

Put the apricots, wine, water and apple juice in a heavy-based saucepan. Add the cloves, nutmeg, cinnamon stick and honey and simmer gently for 30 minutes. Using a sharp knife, cut the top and bottoms off the oranges and lemon, then cut the skin away from the fruit. Thinly slice the oranges and lemon (remove any pips), add the slices to the saucepan with the apricots and continue to cook for 10 minutes. Leave to cool and refrigerate. Serve the fruit compôte in tall glasses, spoon the yogurt on top and dust with cinnamon.

Strawberry soup

This is for those lazy days when you fancy a decadent breakfast in the garden (or in bed).

Serves: 4
Preparation time: 5 minutes

450 g/1 lb strawberries, hulled and roughly chopped
splash dry white wine
450 ml/ ¾ pint live yogurt
large handful fresh mint leaves

Put the strawberries into a food processor, liquidise until smooth, and add a dash of wine. Spoon a dollop or two of thick, creamy yogurt on to the top and scatter over a few fresh mint leaves.

Top tip:

Live yogurt helps to promote a healthy intestinal flora in the gut.

Blueberry buttermilk pancakes

Blueberries contain a high concentration of compounds in their skin that can destroy harmful bacteria in the digestive tract and help to keep it clean and healthy. Make these pancakes and serve with more fresh blueberries.

Serves: 4
Preparation time: 10 minutes
Cooking time: 20 minutes

15 g/½ oz unsalted butter
1 egg
284 ml carton buttermilk
125 g/4 oz unbleached white flour
pinch sea salt flakes
1 tsp baking soda
1 tsp vegetable oil
1 large banana, chopped
handful pecans, toasted and chopped
1 tsp vegetable oil
100 g/7 oz blueberries

Melt the butter in a small saucepan over a medium heat. In a mixing bowl, briskly whisk the egg, buttermilk and melted butter together. In a separate bowl, combine the dry ingredients; mix until blended, then stir into the buttermilk mixture until the dry ingredients are moistened. The batter will be lumpy. Stir the banana and pecans into the batter. Heat a heavy-based frying pan, add the vegetable oil and reduce to a medium heat. Spoon 3 tablespoons of batter for each pancake into the pan. Put a few blueberries on to each pancake and cook until the batter breaks on top (about 2–3 minutes). Turn over and cook until lightly browned, about 1 minute. Keep warm in a low oven on sheets of greaseproof paper, while you cook the others.

Top tip:

Buttermilk was originally nothing more than the tart liquid left after butter was churned. Now buttermilk is a low fat or skimmed milk that is clotted and soured with bacteria cultures (usually lactobacillus). It helps to add a nice sharp flavour and light texture to the pancakes.

Raspberry and blackberry purée

Serves: 2
Preparation time: 5 minutes

450 g/1 lb blackberries
250 g/9 oz raspberries

Mash the two fruits together with a fork and use to top cereals, porridge and yogurts.

Cold fruit compôte

This is so easy, just throw everything together in the evening and leave to soak overnight. At breakfast time, enjoy large servings of this on yogurt or cereal.

Serves: 4
Preparation time: 5 minutes

350 g/12 oz dried fruit, apricots, apples, prunes, pears and figs
200 ml/7 fl oz orange juice
1 cinnamon stick or ½ tsp ground cinnamon
200 ml/7 fl oz apple juice

Roughly chop the fruit and put into a saucepan. Add all of the other ingredients, then bring to the boil. Remove from the heat and leave to cool.

Top tip:

Make sure when you are buying dried fruit that it has not been dipped in glucose (figs, banana chips, pineapple can be).

Blackcurrant purée with yogurt

When blackcurrants are in season, between June and August, this is a must. Eaten hot or cold they are delicious lightly cooked and puréed then swirled through thick creamy yogurt.

Serves: 2
Preparation time: 5 minutes

450 g/1 lb blackcurrants
pinch golden caster sugar, to taste

To prepare the blackcurrants, wash and pull the fruit away from the stalks with a fork. Cook with a little sugar and a couple of tablespoons of water (the fruit produce quite a lot of their own juice). Remember they only need a small amount of cooking time to become soft.

Top tip:

Blackcurrants have a high vitamin C content, and therefore powerful antioxidant properties – it's not surprising that they were once described as 'a fruit favouring longevity'.

Mango purée

This is delicious served on top of muesli or with a spoon of granola. You really need to allow one mango and one orange per person. This is also delicious as a snack served drizzled over a fruit sorbet.

Serves: 2
Preparation time: 10 minutes

2 mangoes
juice of 2 oranges

Cut the mango in half widthways. Twist and separate the halves and remove the stone, as you would do with a peach. Scoop out the flesh from the skin and put into a food processor. Add the orange juice and whizz until smooth.

Berry toasts

Wild blackberries ripen from August to November and traditionally, blackberries were married with the early windfalls. Here, blackberries are mixed with cherries and grated apples to make a purée. Spread it on to thin slices of granary toast – it beats any jam.

Serves: 2–3
Preparation time: 5 minutes

2 apples (preferably Cox's)
large handful cherries
125 g/4 oz blackberries
granary toast

Cut the apples in half, remove the core and grate into a bowl. Cut the cherries in half and stone, add to the apple with the blackberries and mix together. Taste and check that the fruit are sweet enough (try to avoid adding sugar). Spread thickly on to granary toast and enjoy.

Top tip:

Blackberries need to be soft before they will taste sweet.

Bananas with cinnamon on toast

Bananas are a true friend: they are an excellent aid to digestion and the rich potassium supply gives a real boost to our body's maintenance programme. Try always to reach for a banana instead of a biscuit if you are looking for energy.

Serves: 2
Preparation time: 5 minutes

2 slices wholewheat bread
2 bananas
cinnamon, to sprinkle

Lightly toast the bread until pale golden and warm. Peel the banana and squash the fruit on to the toast. Sprinkle lightly with cinnamon, to taste.

Top tip:

Bananas are high in potassium, antioxidant vitamins and rich in pectin, which is a good source of fibre.

Porridge

Porridge is packed with carbohydrate and energy. There are an incredible number of ways to make porridge, quite amazing really when you consider that there are only three main ingredients that make up this dish. As a general rule, for one serving you will need at least ½ cup oats to 1½ cups liquid. If you have friends around for brunch this recipe is quick to prepare and always well received.

Serves: 4
Preparation time: 5 minutes
Cooking times: 10 minutes

185 g/6½ oz organic porridge oats
750 ml/1¼ pint organic milk
750 ml/1¼ pint water
pinch of salt (optional)

Put the milk and water into a saucepan, add the oats and a pinch of salt (optional). Bring to the boil, reduce to a simmer and cook for 5 minutes.

Top tip:

Oats are high in slow-release complex carbohydrates and soluble fibre. Oats are also a good source of B vitamins, iron, zinc and a little vitamin E. Eat oats and you are doing your arteries a real favour as they supply plenty of silicon for healthy artery walls.

Muesli – Bircher style

This dish, based on whole oats, grains, nuts, milk and fruit, was first invented by Dr Bircher-Benner, a Swiss physician and pioneer of food reform. Unlike most shop-bought mueslis, the oats are soaked in milk or water before being mixed with the other ingredients. The result is the oats are slightly creamy with a soft almost cooked texture. You can change the type of fruit depending on what's in season. Alternatively, try my recipe for Spiced muesli.

Serves: 1
Preparation time: 5 minutes (plus soaking overnight – optional)

1 tbsp oats
3 tbsp water or milk to cover oats
live yogurt and honey, to taste
juice of ½ lemon
1 peach or fresh strawberries
1 small apple
125 g/4 oz toasted chopped nuts, such as almonds, walnuts, cashew nuts, hazelnuts

Put the oats and water (or milk) into a bowl and leave to soak overnight (if you prefer a slight crunch, mix them just a short time before you are ready to eat). Stir in yogurt and honey (to taste) and lemon juice. Stone the peach and slice into pieces, and halve the strawberries. Grate the apple and quickly mix all of the fruit into the oats. Add the nuts, stir and enjoy.

Warm apricots with ginger

Serves: 3–4
Preparation time: 5 minutes
Cooking time: 5 minutes

150 g/5 oz unsulphured apricots
2.5 cm/1 inch piece of fresh root ginger, peeled and grated

Put the apricots and ginger in a bowl and pour over enough water to cover. Leave to soak overnight. In the morning, simmer for 5 minutes. Serve the syrupy apricots on top of porridge, a bowl of muesli or mixed into a little fresh natural yogurt.

If you are a fruit jam fan, choose brands that are low in sugar and high in fruit; check the labels.

Spiced muesli

Once you have made the cereal, it will keep for a couple of weeks stored in an airtight container and hence provide you with many breakfasts. You can adapt this muesli recipe to suit your own taste, just add nuts and fruit that you particularly enjoy. Try eating your muesli with fresh fruit juice or soya milk.

Serves: 8
Preparation time: 15 minutes
Cooking time: 5 minutes

40 g/1½ oz sunflower seeds
50 g/2 oz almonds, roughly chopped
75 g/3 oz whole almonds or cashew nuts, roughly chopped
50 g/2 oz coconut chips (or shredded coconut)
300 g/11 oz rolled oats
4 tbsp wheatgerm
125 g/4 oz of both dried apricots, chopped and raisins
75 g/3 oz dried cranberries or blueberries
pinch freshly grated nutmeg and
½ tsp cinnamon
apple juice (or milk) and fresh fruit, to serve

Dry fry the seeds and nuts in a frying pan over a medium heat, stirring constantly, until they begin to brown. Transfer to a bowl. Dry fry the coconut chips for a minute until golden, then add to the bowl of seeds and nuts. Add all of the other ingredients to the bowl and mix everything together. Serve with apple juice or milk and fresh fruit.

Top tip:

For a very quick breakfast to eat on the run, mix about 30 g (1½ oz) of this muesli with 1 small papaya and 1 kiwi (both peeled and cubed). Spoon into a little pot. Take a pot of yogurt and mix the two together.

Granola

Granola is best described as a toasted muesli that is packed with flavour. Eat it on its own or mix it with milk, fruit juice, natural yogurts and/or poached or chopped fresh fruit. You could even use this as a crumble topping or on top of baked apples. So if you find yourself with a little time, make this mixture and keep it in a bag in the freezer for those occasions when you need to make a pudding, quickly.

Makes: about 10 portions
Preparation time: 10 minutes
Cooking time: 35–45 minutes

350 g/12 oz oats
50 g/2 oz wheat germ
50 g/2 oz coconut chips or shredded coconut
50 g/2 oz sesame seeds
75 g/3 oz sunflower seeds
75 g/3 oz cashews or almonds
125 ml/4 fl oz organic olive oil
75 ml/3 fl oz organic runny honey
½ tsp vanilla extract
175 g/6 oz dried fruit, such as apples, apricots, dates, prunes or raisins, chopped into bite-sized pieces.

Preheat the oven to 150°C/300°F/gas mark 2. Grease a rectangular tin. In a large bowl mix the oats, wheat, coconut, sesame seeds, sunflower seeds and nuts.

In a large saucepan combine oil, honey and vanilla. Cook over a gentle heat until the honey is melted.

Pour the wet ingredients over the dry ingredients and mix thoroughly. Spread the mixture out in the tin. Bake for 35–45 minutes, stirring the mixture every 10 minutes. Cool, add the dried fruit. Store in an airtight container.

Top tip:

Have fun making layered breakfast parfaits to eat on the run.

Take a plastic cup with a lid, spoon half of the yogurt (organic natural or fruit), followed by half of the granola and half of the fruit (of your choice). Repeat with the rest of the ingredients and seal with the lid.

Buttermilk oats with fruit and nuts

I had to include this version of porridge for my father. Being the Grant family, we have some Scottish blood in us somewhere and this is an example of an ancient Scottish dish of brose, uncooked porridge. Oats are mixed with hot or cold liquid before adding other ingredients. My suggestions for other ingredients are exactly that, suggestions – add your own selection of fruit and nuts to suit your taste.

Serves: 4
Preparation time: 10 minutes (plus chilling overnight)

50 g/2 oz rolled oats
250 ml/9 fl oz buttermilk
250 ml/9 fl oz organic milk or water
a pinch of salt
2 apples (preferably Cox's)
handful dried blueberries (or raisins)
50 g/2 oz nuts of your choice, such as hazelnuts, toasted and roughly chopped
honey, to taste

Put the oats into a bowl, add the buttermilk, milk (or water) and a pinch of salt. Cover and refrigerate overnight. In the morning, core the apple and grate into a bowl. Add the blueberries or raisins to the apple with the toasted nuts and mix everything together. Stir the fruit mixture into the oats, thin the mixture with a little extra buttermilk, if necessary, and sweeten to taste with honey.

Poached free-range eggs served with fresh spinach

If you keep breakfast egg recipes simple and quick there are so many things that you can do with them.

Serves: 6
Preparation time: 20 minutes
Cooking time: 10 minutes

6 free-range eggs
150 g/5 oz asparagus (optional)
150 g/5 oz baby spinach leaves
2 tbsp balsamic vinegar
4 tbsp extra virgin olive oil
sea salt flakes, freshly ground black pepper

Poach the eggs; put the frying pan over a gentle heat, add boiling water and bring up to a gentle simmer. Break the eggs, one at a time, into the water and let them barely simmer for 1 minute. Turn off the heat and leave to cook for another 9 minutes. Meanwhile, bring a pan of water to the boil, add the asparagus and cook until tender, but still with a bite. Divide the spinach between four plates and top each with a poached egg. Rest asparagus tips around the egg. Mix together the balsamic vinegar and oil, season well and drizzle over the top and around each egg.

Top tip:

Eggs are a fabulous natural fast food, packed with protein, vital minerals including iron and zinc and vitamins.

Omelettes

This is a breakfast idea for when you have a little more time, or you can serve as a brunch.

A group of friends and I spent ten days skiing in a place near Chamonix, called Les Houchées. We were completely spoilt for the whole time during our stay by the couple running the chalet, a fabulous girl, Gina and her talented chef boyfriend, Clint. I was so inspired by some of the dishes Clint served during our stay, that I asked for a few recipes for this book and this is one of them. Remember to use your best omelette pan (we need a base of about 15 cm/6 inches in diameter). This omelette recipe serves one – omelettes are so quick to cook and easy to make, it is better to make them individually.

Serves: 1
Preparation time: 10 minutes
Cooking time: 5 minutes

2 or 3 free-range eggs
30 ml/1½ fl oz single cream
sea salt flakes, freshly ground black pepper
7 g/¼ tsp butter
½ tsp olive oil

Break the eggs into a bowl, add the cream and seasoning and whisk until blended. Heat the butter and oil to as high a heat as you dare. Pour the eggs into the pan, tilting the pan to cover the base. Use a spoon to start to draw the egg from the sides to the middle, so the liquid egg runs into the space, tilting the pan from side to side as you go. Continue until the egg is cooked and there is just a little wet egg on the top. Scatter over your chosen filling (see below), then pop under the grill for a minute or two. Flip the omelette from one side to the centre. Flip again on to a plate and serve.

Top tip:

For fabulous filling ideas try –

- *Brie, tomato chutney and diced avocado*
- *Tomato, coriander, red onion and chilli*
- *Potato, mushrooms and bacon*
- *Fried onion, cooked sausage, tomato slices and Camembert*
- *Red Leicester, peppers and tomato chutney*
- *Feta, spinach and cooked bacon*

Scrambled eggs with herbs and smoked salmon

There is nothing quite so decadent as scrambled eggs with smoked salmon for a relaxing brunch menu. If you are fortunate enough to be making this dish during the chive season (late spring to late autumn) you may find some pretty chive flowers. When you serve this scrambled egg, scatter a few pretty flowers over the top. I tend to use a wooden fork when making scrambled eggs so that I can get right into the corners of the pan and prevent the eggs from sticking.

Serves: 2–3 people
Preparation time: 5 minutes
Cooking time: about 5 minutes

6 free-range eggs
sea salt flakes, freshly ground black pepper
40 g/1½ oz butter
25 g/1 oz Gruyère cheese
handful fresh herbs, such as tarragon, chives, Italian parsley, roughly chopped
chive blossoms to sprinkle over the top (if available)
smoked salmon, to serve
chive blossoms to sprinkle over the top (if available)

Put the eggs into a bowl, whisk for a few minutes, and add a good seasoning of salt and pepper. Melt the butter in a heavy-based saucepan; when hot (the butter should be starting to foam) add the eggs and stir gently to cook evenly. When the eggs are half cooked, add the cheese and herbs and cook for a minute longer. Once the eggs are three-quarters cooked, remove from the heat (the eggs will carry on cooking in the heat of the pan). Once all of the liquid has gone, spoon on to three plates. Serve with strips of smoked salmon and chive blossoms scattered over the top.

Banana and bran muffins

The key to success with this recipe depends on the ripeness of the bananas. You need the fruit to be really ripe so that the flavour is strong enough to come through the finished muffin. The muffin mixture will appear to be quite thin but don't panic. Just get it straight into the tins and into the oven. To check that the muffins are cooked, insert a toothpick into the centre of a muffin and it should come out clean.

Makes: 12
Preparation time: 20 minutes
Cooking time: 20–25 minutes

225 g/8 oz bran cereal
175 g/6 oz oat bran
225 g/8 oz whole wheat flour
2 tsp bicarbonate of soda
1 tsp cinnamon
2 large bananas or 3 small bananas, mashed
a pinch salt
2 eggs, beaten
250 ml/9 fl oz buttermilk
75 ml/3 fl oz honey
125 ml/4 fl oz vegetable oil

Preheat the oven to 200°C/400°F/gas mark 6. Butter the muffin tins or use paper cases. In a large bowl, combine the brans, flour, bicarbonate, cinnamon and salt. In another bowl, mix the beaten eggs, buttermilk, honey and oil. Add the mashed bananas, then add the wet ingredients to the dry ingredients. Mix well but do not beat. Divide into muffin tins. Bake for 20–25 minutes, then leave to set in the tins for 5 minutes before turning out. Cool on a wire rack for 5 minutes before serving.

Top tip:

Muffins are best eaten on the day they are baked. However, do not despair, you do not need to sit and munch your way through lots of muffins, as they freeze really well. Simply leave to cool, put into freezer bags, pushing out any air, seal and freeze. This way you can just take out one at a time, but remember to allow about 10 minutes to thaw.

Kippers with parsley and pepper

If you are looking for a source of protein for breakfast, but you do not feel like eating eggs, why not try kippers? Oily fish such as kippers are rich in vitamins A and D (vitamin D is essential for the absorption of calcium for the development of strong bones and teeth). There is no correct way to cook kippers for breakfast, it is more a matter of taste. If you have never cooked kippers before, it is worth remembering that grilling the fish will intensify its flavour and give it a slight crust. Poaching, on the other hand, tends to lessen the flavour, but will make it more succulent.

Serves: 4
Preparation time: 10 minutes
Cooking time: 3 minutes

4 fresh plump kipper fillets
handful flat leaf parsley, roughly chopped
freshly ground black pepper

Bring a large pan of water to the boil. Add the kippers, return to the boil and remove from the heat. Leave for 3 minutes, drain well. Serve immediately with lots of fresh parsley and freshly ground black pepper scattered over the top.

Top tip:

Try to choose plump, iridescent golden fish with no artificial colouring. Bright orange kippers should be avoided, as this usually means that they have been artificially coloured.

2

Mid-morning boosts

Mid-morning boosts

Eating regularly helps to stabilise your blood sugar levels, so try not to leave more than three to four hours between meals and snacks. This will help to prevent your blood sugar level from getting too low, keep your energy level even and help you refrain from overeating at mealtimes. Tempting as it is to grab a bar of chocolate or a packet of crisps, these will only provide you with short-term energy. Try to keep a few healthy snacks like dried fruits and energy bars with you so that you do not have to rush around trying to find one. This section should provide you with a few other tasty ideas.

As a rule, it is not a good idea to go for long periods without eating: when you eventually eat, the stomach will have to cope with digesting large amounts of food. In addition, an empty stomach can harm the digestive system, leaving it exposed to acids produced in the stomach; the production of digestive juices also slows down over a period of time.

Many people believe their choice of snack is largely dependent on the availability of food. Chocolate, sweets, biscuits and cakes are all very easy to access from machines at work, corner shops and little kiosks. I am sure that convenience plays a major part, yet with just a little effort, you can choose healthy foods that will satisfy your hunger and provide you with a sustained amount of energy. Once you start to choose and enjoy healthy snacks, it will become second nature.

Quick snack ideas

Fruity ideas

- Cut ripe nectarines in half, sprinkle with 1 tablespoon of unrefined sugar and grill for a minute or two, until slightly golden on top. Nectarines, more than peaches, are rich in carotenoids and flavonoids, which serve as antioxidants.
- Slice fresh peaches into a bowl, drizzle with a little lemon juice and scatter over a few fresh torn basil leaves.
- Eat a handful of fresh almonds with a sliced ripe peach and a few raspberries.
- Cut a mango in half widthways, twist to separate the halves and scoop out the stone, like you would a peach. Drizzle with lime juice and eat with a spoon.
- Put the flesh of a mango and the juice of an orange into a food processor and purée until smooth. Serve the purée on top of fresh or frozen yogurt. Freeze any left over in ice cube trays and thaw when needed.
- Cut a grapefruit in half, sprinkle over a little sugar and pop under a hot grill for just under a minute, until caramelised.
- Eat slices of fresh melon which aids rejuvenation as it rushes through the system. Melons are best eaten on their own and are great for cleansing the body of impurities.
- The flesh of watermelon is high in beta-carotene and vitamin C, while the seeds are high in vitamin E and in antioxidant minerals like zinc and selenium. Blend the flesh and seeds into a drink.
- Grapes help to stimulate the metabolism and are a good source of vitamins and minerals.
- Cut a kiwi fruit in half and scoop out the flesh, in much the same way as you would a boiled egg. These little fruit contain twice as much vitamin C as oranges, more fibre than apples and as much vitamin E as avocados.
- Fill lolly containers with fresh fruit juices and freeze. Alternatively, mix yogurt with honey and fresh fruit, blend together and freeze in lolly containers.
- Slice oranges and strawberries and layer. Sprinkle over freshly grated black pepper, which really brings out their flavours.

Nutty ideas

- Eat a handful of dried fruit and nuts, such as sultanas, peanuts, figs, dates, prunes and apricots. These complex carbohydrates give a long lasting release of energy.
- Chop up dates and nuts and mix into yogurt. Nuts contain concentrated sources of body building protein and are rich in natural oils. Nuts are more difficult to digest than fruit, so chop them up and mix with yogurts.
- Almonds, an excellent source of protein, fat, minerals and vitamins, are delicious served with apricots.
- Sunflower seeds are packed with nutrients, including vitamins, minerals, unsaturated fats and protein. Eat on their own or sprinkled into yogurt.

Top tips:

Eat small snacks; if you eat large quantities, your blood supply is diverted to the workload in the digestive tract and away from the brain. That's why a big business lunch can leave you feeling sleepy and sluggish.

You may feel hungry and tired, when all your body really needs is a drink. Harvard research shows that the power of smell has a strong influence on mental alertness. Try to drink peppermint and lemon teas as well as plenty of water.

Eat lots of fresh fruit as snacks.

Eat vitamin B1 or thiamin-rich foods, such as whole grains and fortified foods. B1 gets used up quickly, and when stores become low cognitive problems develop.

Warm and fruity

Rhubarb and ginger compôte

Look out for forced rhubarb from January and garden rhubarb from March. Forced is best cooked for a short time, garden for longer.

Serves: 6
Preparation time: 10 minutes
Cooking time: 10 minutes

450 g/1 lb rhubarb
juice of 1 orange
2 tbsp golden caster sugar
2 pieces stem ginger, finely chopped

Cut the rhubarb into small chunks and put into a saucepan with the orange juice, the golden caster sugar and half of the chopped stem ginger. Bring to simmering point, cover loosely and simmer for 8 minutes. Put the rhubarb into a food processor and whizz until smooth. Add the rest of the ginger and serve.

Top tip:

This takes no time to prepare and cook, so I have suggested making a larger quantity than you need so that you can freeze the rest in ice cube trays. Take a couple of cubes from the freezer as and when needed, leave to thaw and mix into yogurts.

Crispy bread with plums on top

You can make this snack using peaches or nectarines instead of plums.

Serves: 2
Preparation time: 10 minutes
Cooking time: 15–20 minutes

4 ripe plums
4 slices rich dark fruit and whole wheat bread
1 tbsp soft brown sugar
knob butter

Preheat oven to 200°C/400°F/gas mark 5. Halve the plums and remove the stones. Cut the slices of bread and put into a buttered gratin dish. Sprinkle with half of the sugar and place the plums, cut side up, onto the bread. Sprinkle with the rest of the sugar and dot with butter. Bake for 15–20 minutes or until the bread is crisp.

Top tip:

It is important to vary the types of bread that you eat. Slimmers may benefit from eating rye or pumpernickle breads – the darker, heavier, natural European types – rather than the usual whole wheat because wheat contains a high percentage of gluten, which can clog the intestines.

Warm berry and currant salad

The perfect snack for during the summer months when the berries are in season. I have developed the recipe for four people, rather than two, to justify using such a selection of wonderful fruit. If you only want to make the snack for one or two, simply choose a couple of fruits to go with the currants. This is fabulous drizzled while still warm over cold orange sorbet.

Serves: 4
Preparation time: 10 minutes
Cooking time: 5 minutes

2 peaches or nectarines
225 g/8 oz redcurrants
125 g/4 oz blueberries
125 g/4 oz raspberries
125 g/4 oz strawberries
sugar, to taste

Cut the peaches (or nectarines) in half, stone and slice. Put the rest of the fruit and sugar into a stainless steel saucepan with 2 tbsp of water. Bring slowly to the boil. When the currants start to burst and flood the pan with colour, add the other fruit. Simmer for 1 minute (no longer). Serve while still warm with soya yogurt.

Honeyed pears

I hope you will agree that most of the snack ideas in this section are very quick to make and use accessible ingredients. This recipe is another example of just that.

Serves: 2
Preparation time: 5 minutes
Cooking time: 5 minutes

4 ripe pears
25 g/1 oz butter
2 tbsp honey
thick yogurt, to serve (optional)

Core the pears and cut into bite-sized chunks. Melt the butter in a pan, add the pears and cook for about 5 minutes, until the pears are starting to go golden around the edges. Drizzle over the honey and serve with or without yogurt.

Top tip:

Pears are a mild diuretic and laxative and they contain lots of vitamins and minerals.

Hot bananas

There are many mid-morning boosts that can be prepared using bananas.

Serves: 2
Preparation time: 5 minutes
Cooking time: 5 minutes

2 bananas
juice of 1 orange
2 tbsp honey
handful hazelnuts, toasted and roughly chopped

Slice the bananas in half lengthways and rest on a baking tray. Drizzle over the orange juice and brush with honey. Grill for 5 minutes, until the bananas turn golden brown. Scatter over the nuts, pushing them into the fruit and serve.

Top tip:

Banana lollies make excellent snacks if you are looking for snacks for older children (but always check for nut allergies first). Roll bananas in orange juice and then in chopped and toasted nuts, push a lolly stick into the bottom of each banana and freeze.

Hot oranges with crushed cardamom

It is great if you can get into the habit of appreciating the natural sweetness of fruit, but here you may like to add a sprinkling of soft brown sugar to the fruit.

Serves: 2
Preparation time: 10 minutes
Cooking time: 10–15 minutes

2 cardamom pods
3 oranges
2 bananas
orange flower water

Preheat oven to 200°C/400°F/gas mark 6. Remove the small black seeds from the cardamom pods and crush with a pestle and mortar. Cut four squares of foil. Slice the tops and bottoms off the oranges, then peel the fruit working your way around with a sharp knife. Cut the orange into segments and place on the foil. Peel and slice the bananas, then add to the orange. Sprinkle with a little orange flower water and the cardamom seeds. Wrap the foil around the fruit and secure at the top. Bake for 10–15 minutes. Eat while still warm with a scoop of Orange and passion fruit sorbet (see page 166) and a drizzle of passion fruit over the top.

Cold and fruity

Berry and apple sundae

We eat with our eyes, I do believe that. If the food looks good, we are far more likely to enjoy eating it. This snack looks so pretty served in glasses, it is always a joy to eat. For an alternative to nuts on the top, sprinkle over Granola (see page 53).

Serves: 2
Preparation time: 10 minutes

150 g/5 oz blackberries, blueberries or raspberries
3 Bramley or Cox's apples
150 ml/5 fl oz Greek yogurt
2 tbsp honey
125 g/4 oz hazelnuts, toasted and chopped

Pop a few berries in the bottom of two glasses. Core and grate the apple (mix with a little lemon juice if you are not going to eat this straight away) and sprinkle over the berries. Spoon over some yogurt and a little drizzle of honey. Repeat layers starting with more berries. Finish with chopped and toasted hazelnuts.

Top tips:

The supermarkets are reinstating many native varieties of apples alongside an increasingly large range of imported. Sweet-flavoured Discovery start the British season in August, followed by Worcester Pearmain in September to October. Egremont Russett are nutty flavoured and rough skinned and appear from October to December, with my favourite, Cox's Orange Pippin, available from October through to January. Not to forget the Chiver's Delight from November to January and the aromatic fruit of D'Arcy Spice, which is around from January to April.

If you are using a corer, core the apple before peeling to prevent the fruit from cracking.

Things on toast

Roasted pepper and vegetable soup with homemade sea salt and rosemary flat breads

Fresh tuna Niçoise

Vegetarian sushi

Apple spread for malt loaf

Grab a fresh malt loaf to nibble on when you get hungry. Instead of piling on the butter, make a very quick apple spread. If you feel like a bit of a treat, add a splash of Calvados instead of the honey.

Serves: 2
Preparation time: 10 minutes

3 ripe apples (preferably Cox's)
pinch ground cinnamon
1 tsp honey

Peel, core and chop the apple, then put the flesh into a bowl. Mash the apple to a purée. Add the cinnamon and honey and mix together.

Top tip:

I was fortunate enough to experience the wonders of a spice trail in Zanzibar. It was here that I saw rows and rows of trees where the cinnamon bark comes from. Where possible, use the whole fresh cinnamon bark, unless you are looking for a quick easy burst of flavour as we are in this recipe.

Intense berry fool

This really is intense, especially when you add a rich berry or fruity liqueur. Use as a sauce to swirl though thick creamy yogurt, or over a good-quality sorbet, frozen yogurt or ice cream.

Serves: 2
Preparation time: 5 minutes

250 g/8 oz raspberries, strawberries or blackberries (or a combination of all three)
1–2 tsp golden caster sugar
juice of ½ lemon
1 tbsp fruit liqueur, such as crème de cassis or framboise

Put the raspberries, strawberries or blackberries into a food processor and purée until smooth. Add golden caster sugar and lemon juice to taste. Flavour with the liqueur of your choice. Strain through a sieve.

Top tip:

Raspberries are known for having excellent uplifting properties and are a good source of vitamins and minerals.

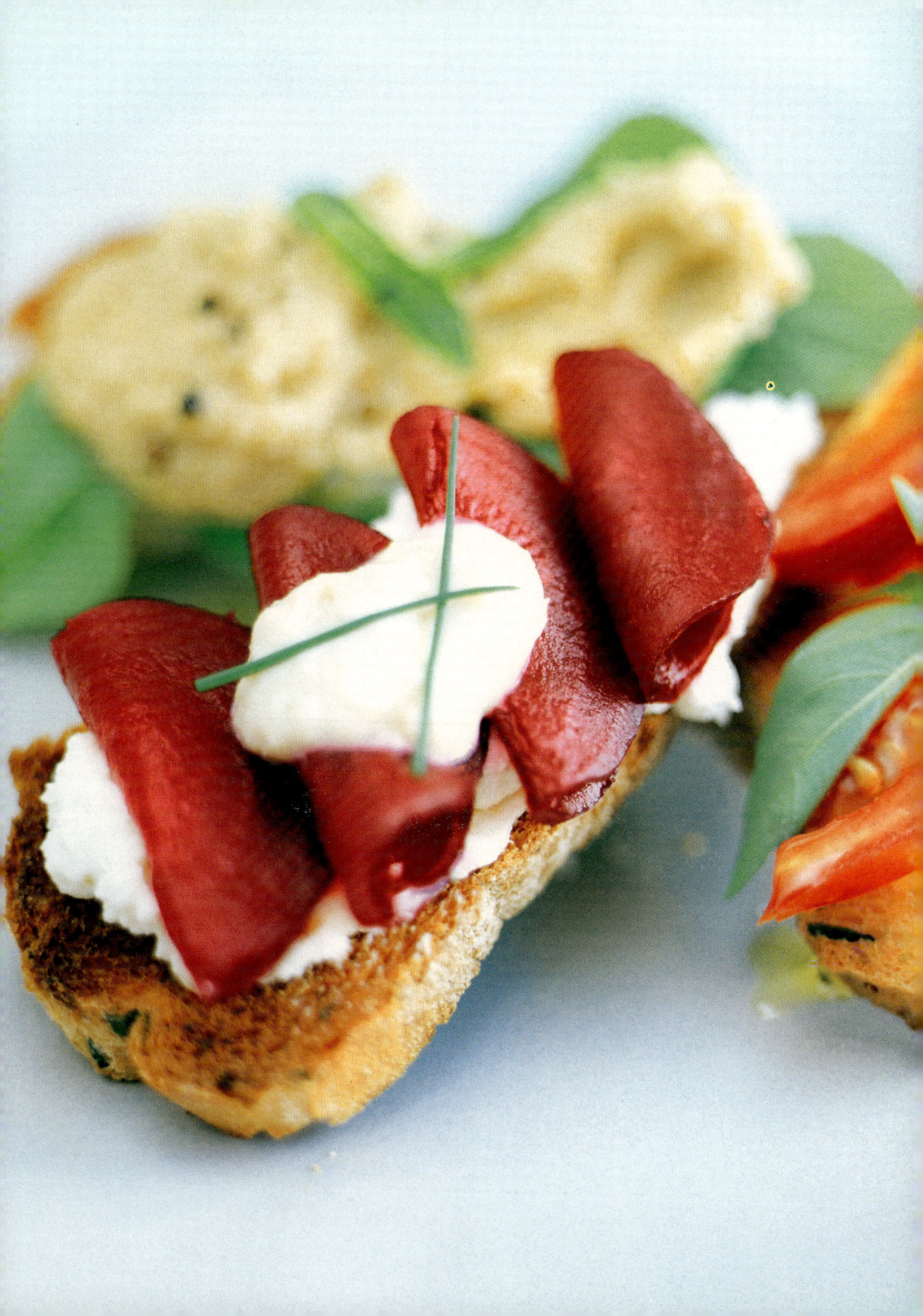

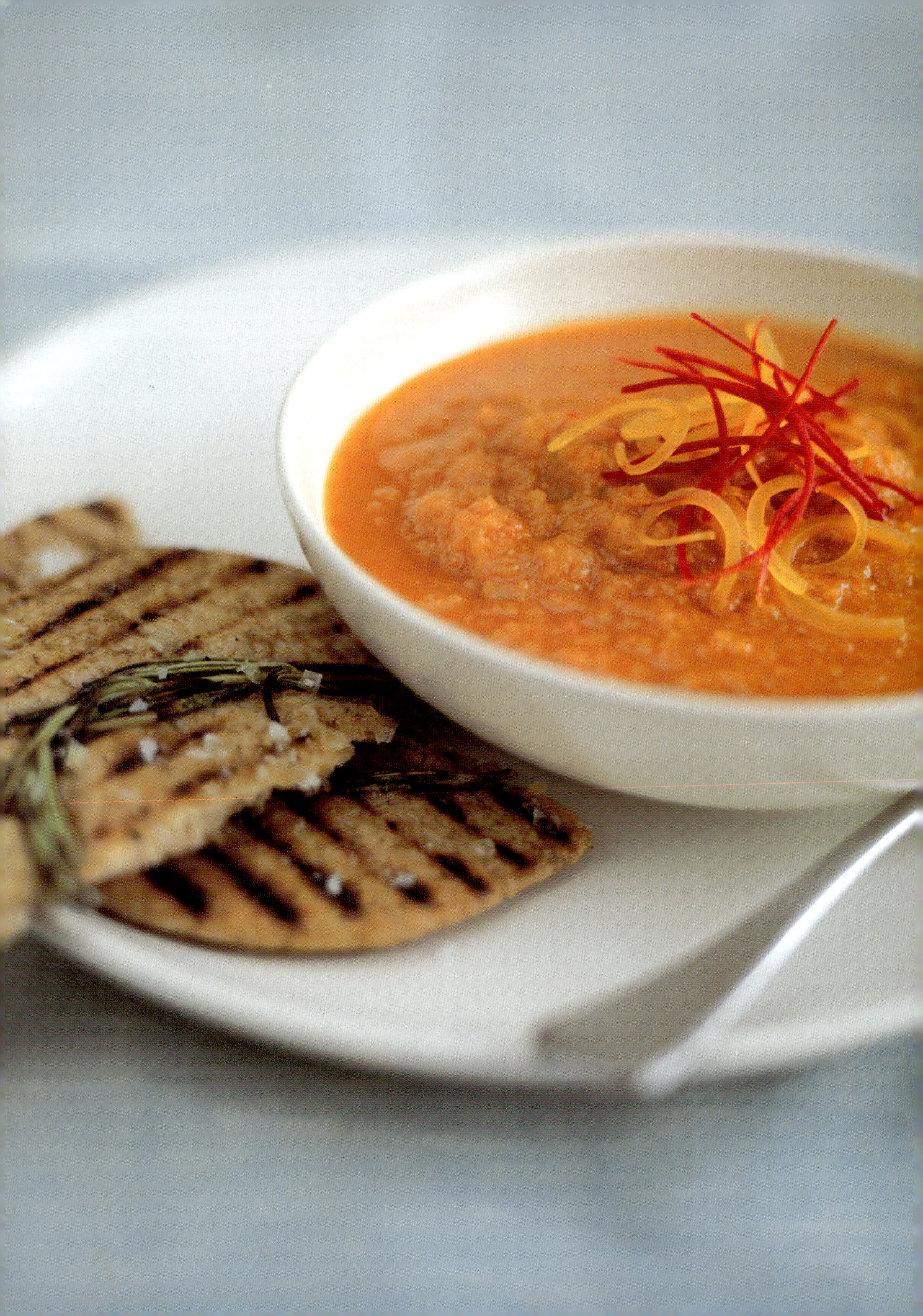

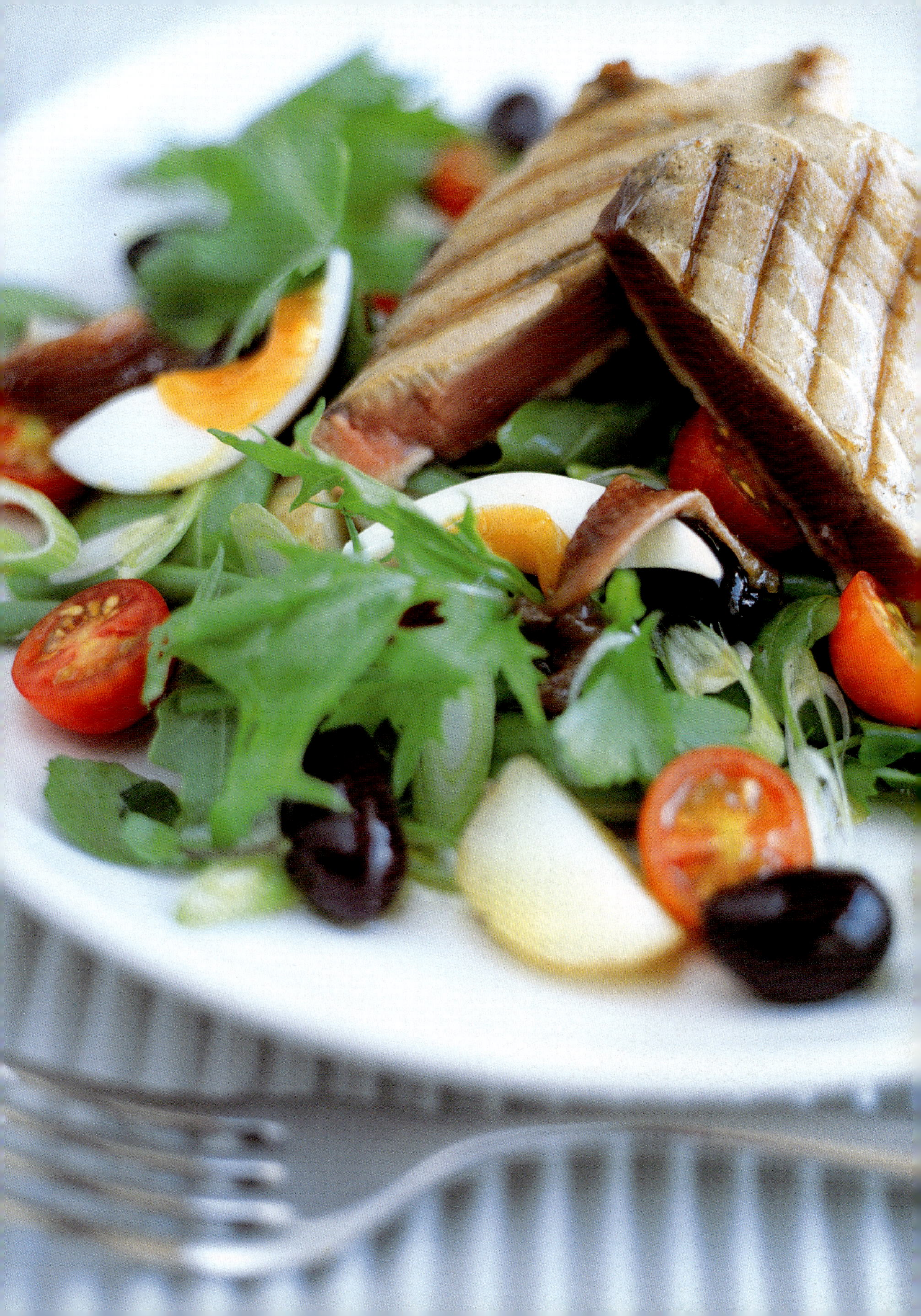

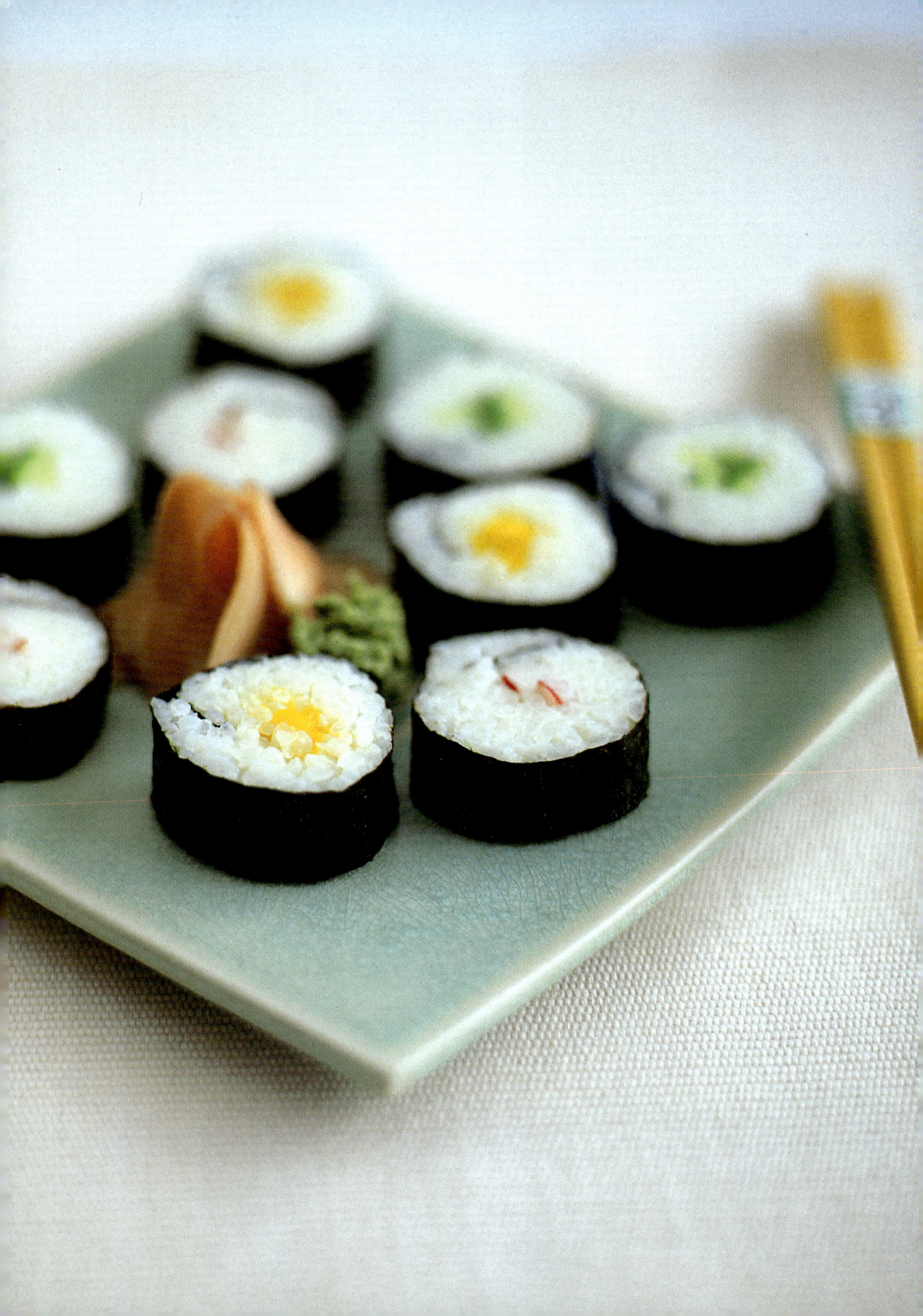

Mango and lychees with ginger

It is amazing how something as simple as the addition of ginger can transform a bowl of fresh fruit.

Serves: 2
Preparation time: 10 minutes

1 mango or papaya
125 g/4 oz fresh pineapple
6 fresh lychees
2 pieces stem ginger, finely chopped
zest of ½ lime
1 tbsp ginger syrup

Peel and stone (or seed) the mango (or papaya), cut the flesh into bite-sized cubes and put into a bowl. Peel the pineapple and cut the flesh into cubes. Peel and stone the lychees and add to the fruit. Stir in the ginger and lime zest, drizzle over the ginger syrup and serve.

Top tip:

Fresh root ginger steeped in hot water is a drink that I love at the beginning of the day. Fresh ginger aids digestion and is therefore an excellent ingredient to incorporate into the daily diet.

Lemon and orange cups with crushed blueberries

Like most homemade ice creams or sorbets, the best texture is achieved when made in an ice cream machine. However, for the best results using a conventional freezer, put this mixture into small containers to encourage the sorbet to freeze quickly and, hence, reduce the size of the ice crystals. This makes a really refreshing treat for the middle of the morning or afternoon.

Serves: 4
Preparation time: 20 minutes (plus freezing time)

9 oranges
2 juicy lemons
honey, to sweeten
250 g/8 oz blueberries

Juice the oranges and combine in a food processor with 2 lemons that have been peeled and quartered. Add enough honey to sweeten. Pour the mixture into ice cube trays, lolly containers or small plastic containers. Freeze for at least 3 hours. If you have frozen the mixture in large containers quickly mix the sorbet or whizz in a food processor to break up the ice crystals before serving.

Crush the blueberries. Spoon the sorbet into little cups, drizzle the crushed blueberries over the middle of each, and serve.

Frozen ice cream crunch with crushed raspberries

This is another successful way to encourage children to eat fresh fruit, but it is also enjoyed by adults. Make up a few and keep in the freezer for those snack attacks.

Serves: 4
Preparation time: 20 minutes

250 g/8 oz Granola (see page 53)
150 g/5 oz whole wheat sweet biscuits, crushed
3 tbsp Mango purée (see page 49)
300 g/10½ oz frozen vanilla soya ice cream (Swedish Glace is good)

for the sauce:
250 g/8 oz raspberries
1 tsp lime juice
1 tsp golden icing sugar

Mix together the granola, biscuits and mango purée. Spoon into paper cases, dot with frozen ice cream, cover and freeze. Push the raspberries through a sieve with a wooden spoon, add the lime juice and golden icing sugar. Serve the little cases with a jug of the sauce for drizzling over the top.

Top tip:

Vary this mixture as much as you like; try with different fruit pureés and frozen yogurts instead of ice cream.

Bars

Apple and toasted hazelnut flapjacks

I think flapjacks are nicest when they are soft, moist and slightly crumbly, not hard and chewy. The secret is to take them out of the oven while they are still slightly soft as they will go crisp as they cool. If you want to vary this recipe, use bananas instead of apples, just make sure that they are really ripe to give the mixture a true banana flavour.

Makes: 12
Preparation time: 20 minutes
Cooking time: 20 minutes

125 g/4 oz butter
75 g/3 oz soft brown sugar
2 tbsp syrup
350 g/12 oz porridge oats
½ tsp baking powder
2 apples, cored and grated
50 g/2 oz hazelnuts, roughly chopped and toasted

Preheat the oven to 180°C/350°F/gas mark 4. Butter a Swiss roll tin (about 23 cm/9 inch x 33 cm/13 inch). Melt the butter, sugar and syrup together in a large saucepan over a low heat. Mix in the oats, baking powder, apples and nuts, then spoon into the tin. Bake for 20 minutes or until the edges are beginning to go golden. Cut into squares while still warm, then allow to cool in the tin before transferring to a wire rack and leave to cool.

Nutty fruity slice

A very easy delicious sticky bar made of oats, nuts, dried fruit, organic honey, syrup, butter and sesame seeds. They are high in iron, calcium, protein and fibre.

Makes: 15
Preparation time: 15 minutes
Cooking time: 20 minutes

100 g/3 oz organic butter
25 g/1 oz golden caster sugar
75 g/3 oz golden syrup
250 g/9 oz jumbo rolled oats
25 g/1 oz sunflower seeds, toasted
50 g/2 oz brazil nuts, chopped and toasted
75 g/3 oz dried apricots and raisins, roughly chopped, or combination of other dried fruits
25 g/1 oz cranberries
1 tbsp sesame seeds, toasted

Grease a 20.5 cm/8 inch square tin. Preheat the oven to 180°C/350°F/gas mark 4. Put the butter, sugar and syrup into a pan and heat until the butter is melted. Add the rest of the ingredients and mix well. Tip into the greased tin, then cook for 25 minutes. Mark into squares and cool in the tin. Cut and store in an airtight container.

Very quick sandwiches/ things on toast

Dates with cream cheese and banana

Serves: 1
Preparation time: 5 minutes

2 slices of wholemeal bread
100 g/3½ oz cream cheese
1 banana
5 dates, stoned

Spread the pieces of bread with cream cheese, slice the banana and rest on top. Roughly chop the dates and scatter over the bananas. Top with the other piece of bread and cut in half.

Bean purée with fresh mint and spinach

Make these rolls or serve the purée with fresh salad and fingers of bread

Serves: 2–3
Preparation time: 10 minutes

420 g can chickpeas, drained and rinsed
1 clove garlic, peeled and crushed
juice of ½ lime
2 tbsp extra virgin olive oil
2 tbsp water
sea salt flakes, freshly ground black pepper
fresh mint leaves, roughly torn
75 g/3 oz baby spinach (or as much as you can pack into the rolls)
2–3 wholemeal rolls

Put the chickpeas, garlic and lime juice in a blender and process until smooth. Gradually add the oil in a thin stream, keeping the motor running. Then add the water and purée until the chickpeas are smooth. Season with salt and freshly ground black pepper. Cut the rolls in half, spread the purée into the middle, scatter over fresh mint leaves and pack each with lots of baby spinach (as much as you can squeeze in).

Egg mayo with cress

Always use organic free-range eggs, as you will notice a difference in taste. Keep the eggs at room temperature and bring the water to the boil before you add them to the pan. The eggs will continue to cook once they have been removed from the pan so make sure that you run them under cold water.

Serves: 2
Preparation time: 15 minutes
Cooking time: 6 minutes

3 free-range eggs
1 tbsp mayonnaise
1 tbsp natural yogurt
sea salt flakes, freshly ground black pepper
4 slices wholemeal or white bread
large handful fresh cress

Bring the water to the boil, add the eggs and boil for 6 minutes. This will give you soft boiled eggs, that is, the yolk will be slightly runny in the centre. If you prefer the yolk to be completely set, boil for 7 minutes instead. Shell the eggs under running cold water and put them into a clean dry bowl. Season and roughly mash with a fork. Leave the egg to cool, add the mayonnaise, natural yogurt and mix together. Spread the egg mayonnaise on 2 slices of bread and scatter over fresh cress. Top with another piece of bread, cut in half and serve.

Herby tomatoes

For those of you not too keen on eating lots of bread, mix the tomatoes with slices of mozzarella and basil, drizzle with olive oil and season.

Serves: 2
Preparation time: 5 minutes

2–3 ripe beef tomatoes
sea salt flakes, freshly ground black pepper
2 slices bread (this would work well with a nutty bread such as walnut bread which is available from many supermarket bakeries)
extra virgin olive oil
handful fresh basil

Cut the tomatoes into thick slices and season well. Brush the bread with oil, heat a griddle pan and cook the bread for a few minutes on each side, until golden and crisp. Pile the tomatoes on to the toasted bread. Drizzle with extra virgin olive oil and scatter over the fresh basil leaves.

Cottage cheese with pineapple

This is really refreshing and is particularly delicious made with a multigrain bread or good wholemeal. Alternatively, eat with fresh salad ingredients.

Serves: 2
Preparation time: 10 minutes

125 g/4 oz cottage cheese
4 slices mixed grain bread
75 g/3 oz fresh pineapple
handful pine nuts, toasted
handful English lettuce leaves, washed and roughly torn
sea salt flakes, freshly ground black pepper

Spread the cottage cheese over 2 slices of the bread, then arrange the pineapple slices over the top. Sprinkle with pine nuts and then arrange the lettuce over the top. Season lightly with salt and pepper and top with the remaining slices of bread.

Beetroot with horseradish

Serves: 2
Preparation time: 10 minutes

150 g/5 oz cooked beetroot (not in vinegar)
4 tbsp cream cheese
2–3 tsps creamed horseradish, to taste
sea salt flakes, freshly ground black pepper
2–3 flat breads

Drain the beetroot and slice thinly. Cream the cream cheese with the horseradish and season to taste. Spread the cheese thickly on to flat breads, then top with the beetroot.

3

Lunches

Lunches

We need to eat our lunch sitting down rather than on the run. Our digestive system needs a plentiful supply of oxygen (brought in by the blood) and the appropriate hormones to enable it to work efficiently. If you do not sit still, oxygen is diverted away from the stomach to other muscles, which hinders digestion and can result in indigestion or stomach cramps. Also we should relax for 10–15 minutes afterwards to counteract the release of hormones that make us feel sleepy after a meal.

We do not want to overload our digestive systems by eating foods that give our bodies a huge task to break down. We need fresh, light foods that are packed with vitamins, minerals and energy, particularly when we have a busy afternoon ahead of us and need to be bright and alert. Lunch is a very important meal of the day so we do need to make sure that we eat a sensible amount, to keep us feeling satisfied during the afternoon.

There are many different ideas here for you to choose from. So if you are looking for soup, a sandwich, a salad (warm or cold) or a more substantial carbohydrate or protein-based dish, take a look at the selection and have fun in the kitchen. There are many recipes here that are quick to prepare in the morning and easy to transport so that you can take them to work.

I have included a large section of fresh salads. With the ever-growing trend towards lighter eating, elaborate salads inspired by the traditional cooking in France or Italy have become popular main courses. The important thing to notice here is just how easy it is to incorporate fresh and raw salad ingredients into your diet. Choose the salads and ingredients that are in season at the time and have fun preparing and eating the wonderful textures and flavours that they provide. Add other ingredients to the salads to suit your tastes.

You may find that some of these recipes are also good for starters.

Have fun in the kitchen and eat life to the full!

Soups

Watercress and potato soup

Serve this creamy hot soup with small bowls of the croûtons. Watercress has been used in cooking since at least the seventeenth century. Whether it was used for pleasure or medicinal purposes is hard to ascertain, since early recipes are few and far between. Today, however, watercress is underused in cooking. Try adding it to mash for a peppery kick or add to stir-fries at the last minute.

Serves: 6
Preparation time: 20 minutes
Cooking time: 25–30 minutes

2 tbsp olive oil
2–3 shallots or cloves garlic, peeled and finely chopped
1 celery stalk, finely sliced
2 large potatoes (450 g/1 lb), peeled and diced
900 ml/1½ pints vegetable stock
bunch fresh oregano leaves, roughly chopped
sea salt flakes, freshly ground pepper
150 g/5 oz watercress, roughly chopped and washed
75 ml/3 fl oz double cream, thick yogurt or soya yogurt
sprigs fresh watercress, washed

for the croûtons:
4 thick slices white bread
2 tbsp olive oil
sea salt flakes, freshly ground black pepper

Preheat the oven to 200°C/400°F/gas mark 6. Heat the oil in a saucepan and fry the shallots and celery until soft and lightly golden (for about 5 minutes). Add the potato and toss to coat in the oil. Add the stock and oregano, bring to the boil and simmer for 15 minutes.

Meanwhile, make the croûtons; cut the slices into big cubes and put on to a baking tray. Drizzle liberally with oil and scatter over salt and freshly ground black pepper. Bake for 10–15 minutes until golden and toasted all over, then put into a serving bowl.

Add the watercress to the soup, transfer to a food processor and whizz until smooth. Pour the soup back into the saucepan and heat through for a couple of minutes. Season to taste, ladle into warm serving bowls and swirl a little of the cream in. Scatter a few croûtons and sprigs of watercress on to each and serve with little bowls of the remaining croûtons.

Top tip:

Watercress provides more vitamin C per mg than oranges. The people of the ancient world knew all about its health-giving properties, hence the story of Zeus eating watercress specifically to overcome his father. Watercress is aquatic and has a peppery flavour.

Chilled gazpacho with spicy cayenne croûtons

Soups do not get simpler than this: even my husband made this and loved it. Of course, he then wondered why it has taken me so long to develop the recipes for this book when they are all so easy!

There are two really cool ways to enjoy this soup, either served with a bowl of spicy crunchy croûtons or a big bunch of fresh, wild rocket leaves piled into the middle of each bowl.

Serves: 4
Preparation time: 20 minutes
Cooking time: 10–15 minutes

4 slices thick granary bread
2–3 tbsp extra virgin olive oil
cayenne and paprika pepper
900 g/2 lb very ripe cherry tomatoes or baby plum tomatoes, roughly chopped
1 cucumber, peeled, seeded and chopped
1 clove garlic, peeled and chopped
1 red chilli, seeded and finely chopped
2 spring onions, finely chopped
4 tbsp extra virgin olive oil
1 tbsp red wine vinegar
1 tbsp golden caster sugar
sea salt flakes
fresh baby rocket leaves, to garnish

Preheat the oven to 180°C/350°F/gas mark 4. Cut the bread into cubes and place on a baking tray. Drizzle with oil and scatter over the cayenne pepper and paprika. Bake for 10–15 minutes, turning frequently until golden and crisp.

Make the soup; put all of the ingredients, except seasoning, into a food processor and whizz until smooth. Season to taste with sea salt flakes and cayenne pepper. Spoon into bowls, top with a sprinkling of paprika, a drizzle of extra virgin olive oil and a big pile of fresh baby rocket leaves. Serve with a big bowl of spicy croûtons.

Top tips:

As a general rule of thumb, the smaller and skinnier the chilli, the hotter it is. Do not rub your eyes after preparing chillies. If your hands are sensitive wear rubber gloves when you are preparing them.

Garlic helps to cleanse the blood and reduce cholesterol and has antibacterial, antifungal and antiviral properties. Garlic should always be used when fresh or it develops a bitter taste. If you want the garlic to be slightly milder in flavour, blanch the cloves (before peeling) for 3–4 minutes in boiling water before using in recipes.

Use stale bread to make croûtons, which you can then pack into freezer bags and freeze until required.

Carrot soup with honey and ginger

Soups do not need to take hours to prepare. Homemade stocks are my first choice for soups, but failing that, use Swiss Vegetable Bouillon Powder. It has a lovely fresh flavour unlike so many of the stock cubes available. For those interested, it is gluten free and there is also a vegan variety. Both types are available from all good supermarkets.

Serves: 4–6
Preparation time: 20 minutes
Cooking time: 20–30 minutes

1.1 kg/2lb 3oz carrots, washed and scraped
2 onions (skin attached)
head of celery, roughly chopped
4 cloves garlic (skin on)
4 tbsp extra virgin olive oil
5 cm/2 inch fresh root ginger, peeled and finely chopped
2–3 tsp ground coriander
1.4 litres/2½ pints vegetable stock
sea salt flakes, freshly ground black pepper
1 tbsp honey, to taste

Preheat the oven to 200°C/400°F/gas mark 6. Roughly chop the carrots and put into a roasting tin. Cut the onion into small wedges (with skin attached), then add to the carrots with the celery and garlic cloves. Drizzle over 3 tablespoons of oil and roast the vegetables for 20–30 minutes, until cooked. Heat the remaining oil in a saucepan, add the ginger and ground coriander, and sauté until the ginger is soft. Remove the skin from the onion, and put the flesh into a food processor. Squeeze the garlic pulp out of their skins into the processor, add the carrots, celery, cooked spices and half of the vegetable stock, then whizz. Transfer to a saucepan, and add enough stock to make the desired consistency. Season with salt, pepper and honey to taste, then serve.

Top tip:

Carrots are so rich in beta-carotene that one or two should supply your vitamin A needs for a whole day. They are also an excellent tonic and rejuvenator.

Pea and lettuce soup

This is the perfect soup to cook during the summer months from mid-July to September when peas are in season. It may take a little while to pod the peas, but it is definitely worth the effort. As a guide, you will need approximately double the weight of peas in their pods in order to get the right weight of shelled peas. If the season for peas has passed, try frozen peas, which incidentally do still have a high nutrient content. Generally, I tend to eat lettuce raw rather than cooked and it is best torn (not cut, as this bruises the leaves). However, the more robust leaves, such as Cos and Romaine, are great added to soups or stir-fries.

Serves: 4
Preparation time: 25–30 minutes
Cooking time: 25 minutes

2 tbsp light and fruity olive oil
1 onion, peeled and chopped
600 ml/1 pint good-quality chicken stock (preferably organic)
600 ml/1 pint water
500 g/1lb 2 oz fresh (shelled) or frozen tiny peas
½ head of Romaine or Cos lettuce
45 g/1½ oz fresh firm mint leaves, roughly chopped
sugar, sea salt flakes, freshly ground black pepper, to taste

thin crispy croûtons (optional, see page 78)

Heat the oil in a saucepan, add the onion and fry for at least 5 minutes, or until cooked and soft. Add the chicken stock and bring up to a simmer, then add the peas. Cook until the peas are tender (this will take 5 minutes), add the lettuce and cook for a few minutes more. Add the mint leaves and season to taste. Serve hot or cold.

Top tips:

As a general rule, the more green the vegetable, the more vitamins and minerals it will contain.

The best way to store lettuce is to keep it attached to the root and seal in a plastic bag before refrigerating. Cut with a sharp knife when preparing to avoid damage and loss of nutrients.

Fennel soup with lemon oil

This is a really refreshing soup: the flavours are quite subtle and the lemon gives the whole dish a little kick. Fennel has a subtle aniseed flavour that becomes slightly more intense with the addition of the tarragon. This soup is great for a lunch, but it is also delicious served as a starter as it provokes and entices the palate ready to enjoy the rest of the meal.

Serves: 4
Preparation time: 15 minutes
Cooking time: 30 minutes

450 g/1 lb leeks
1 large fennel bulb
25 g/1 oz butter
1 tbsp olive oil
1 small onion, peeled and sliced
1.1litres/2 pints vegetable stock
2 tbsp fresh tarragon, roughly chopped
sea salt flakes, freshly ground black pepper
150 ml/¼ pint single cream
juice of ½ lemon

Finely slice the leeks. Cut the fennel in half lengthways and slice into thin strips. Melt the butter with the oil in a saucepan. Add the onion, leeks and fennel and cook over a gentle heat for approximately 10 minutes, until just turning translucent and brown at the edges. Stir frequently. Add the stock, 1 tablespoon of the tarragon and a pinch of salt, bring to the boil and simmer gently until the fennel is soft – approximately 20 minutes. Cool, then blend the soup in a food processor until really smooth. Stir in the cream and the remaining tarragon. Add the lemon juice and season to taste.

Top tips:

Fennel has a sweet liquorice/aniseed flavour and it has a calming and soothing effect on the body.

To prevent fennel from turning brown once prepared, immerse in water with lemon juice.

Tomato soup with garlic and lots of herbs

Make sure that you choose ripe tomatoes with plenty of flavour. As with all recipes, the end result is only as good as the quality of the ingredients used.

Serves: 6
Preparation time: 20 minutes
Cooking time: 35–45 minutes

900 g/2 lb ripe tomatoes
1 whole head garlic
2 onions
3 tbsp extra virgin olive oil
sea salt flakes, freshly ground black pepper
600 ml/1 pint vegetable stock or chicken stock
handful each of fresh basil and parsley, roughly chopped

Preheat oven to 180°C/350°F/gas mark 4. Put the tomatoes into a roasting tin, break the garlic into cloves and add to the tin. Cut the onions into quarters (leave the skin attached) and add to the tomatoes. Drizzle with the oil, season well and roast for 35–45 minutes. Squeeze the garlic out of their skins into a food processor. Peel the onion and add the flesh to the garlic. Peel the tomatoes, add three-quarters of the tomatoes and stock, and whizz until you are happy with the texture (this works really well either smooth or slightly chunky). Transfer to a saucepan, add the reserved tomatoes and warm through. Season to taste. Stir in the fresh herbs and serve.

Roasted pepper and vegetable soup

Roasting vegetables makes their flavour much more intense and concentrates their natural sweetness.

Serves: 4
Preparation time: 15 minutes
Cooking time: 35–45 minutes

1 onion, quartered (skin left on)
3 cloves garlic (skin left on)
2 carrots, halved (scraped)
2 celery sticks, cut into thirds
1 leek, white part, halved
2 yellow peppers, seeded and halved
2 red peppers, seeded and halved
1 red chilli, seeded and chopped
2 tbsp extra virgin olive oil
sea salt flakes, freshly ground black pepper
900 ml/1½ pint–1.1 litres/2 pints vegetable stock
fresh coriander leaves and thin strips of pepper, to serve

Preheat the oven to 200°C/400°F/gas mark 6. Put all of the vegetables into an ovenproof dish, add the chilli and oil, and season well. Roast for 35–45 minutes or until the peppers are soft and cooked. Remove the garlic and onion skin and put all of the vegetables into a food processor. Add half of the stock and whizz until smooth. Transfer to a saucepan and add enough stock to make a consistency that you are happy with. Season to taste and serve.

Thai sweetcorn soup with coconut

To some, seeing sweetcorn on the market stalls may be a sad sign as it signifies the end of summer. I like to think of it as the beginning of a new season, autumn. The short season for corn on the cob begins in August and ends in September. If the weather is good during these months, wrap the cob up in its own husk and cook on the barbeque, serve with dollops of houmous and fresh parsley on top. This soup is so filling it is definitely a complete meal on its own and, more importantly, it is absolutely bursting with flavour.

Serves: 4
Preparation time: 20 minutes
Cooking time: 30 minutes

6 ears fresh corn or 500g/1¼ lb canned sweetcorn
1 large onion, peeled and finely chopped
3 cloves garlic, peeled and crushed
2 cm/1 inch piece fresh root ginger, peeled and finely chopped
1 red chilli, halved, seeded and finely chopped
1 stick lemon grass, outer leaves removed
virgin olive oil, to drizzle
1 large potato, peeled and cut into small chunks
400 ml can coconut milk
300 ml/10 fl oz vegetable stock
4 tbsp fresh coriander, roughly chopped
juice of half a lime

Preheat oven 220°C/450°F/gas mark 8. Peel the corn husks away from each corn and put them into a roasting tin with the onion, garlic, ginger, chilli, lemon grass and potato. Mix well. Drizzle with oil and roast for 25–30 minutes, then leave to cool. If using canned sweetcorn, roast all the other vegetables for 20 minutes before adding the corn to the roasting tin; continue roasting for 10 minutes. Remove the lemon grass from the pan and discard. Scrape the kernels away from the cobs. Put the coconut milk and stock into a large saucepan; add half of the corn and all of the roasted vegetables and spices. Transfer the soup to a food processor and whizz until smooth. Return to the saucepan, add the remaining corn and simmer gently for 5 minutes. Stir in the coriander and lime juice and season to taste.

Top tips:

Lemon grass should be bruised before chopping to release the flavour. Use only the bottom part of the stalks as the top is too tough and fibrous. To store lemon grass put in a plastic bag in the fridge or freezer.

Coconut milk is not that found in the centre of the coconut, it is the juice extracted from the white flesh mixed with water. The remaining white flesh left after extracting the juice is used as desiccated coconut. Coconut cream is desiccated coconut ground to an oily paste, which sets into solid blocks. A homemade version of coconut milk can be made by dissolving a chunk of coconut cream in boiling water.

Italian chickpea soup with pesto

If you can get hold of some young fresh broad beans, add a handful to the soup. For maximum flavour, this pesto is best used the same day it is made. However, it will keep for a couple of days in the fridge, just cover with a thin layer of olive oil and wrap tightly in cling film. Alternatively, use a pesto from a good deli.

Serves: 4
Preparation time: 15 minutes
Cooking time: 50 minutes

4 ripe tomatoes
30 ml/2 tbsp olive oil
2 onions, peeled and finely chopped
2 garlic cloves, peeled and finely chopped
1 leek, finely sliced
2 sprigs fresh rosemary
400 g/14oz can chickpeas, drained
1.2 litres/2 pints vegetable stock
125 g/4 oz peas (need approximately 250 g/8 oz of peas in pods)
125 g/4 oz French beans, halved
1 courgette, diced
2 tbsp chopped fresh parsley
sea salt flakes, freshly ground black pepper

for the pesto:
2–3 cloves garlic, peeled and sliced
40 g/1½ oz pine nuts, chopped
100 g/3½ oz fresh basil
50 ml/2 fl oz extra virgin olive oil
50 g/2 oz Parmesan cheese, grated
sea salt flakes, freshly ground black pepper

Roughly chop the tomatoes. Heat the oil in a large saucepan, add the onion, garlic, leek and rosemary, and fry gently for 10 minutes until softened, but not coloured. Add the chickpeas, stock, tomatoes, peas and beans, bring to the boil and simmer for 10 minutes. Add the courgette and parsley, cook for another 5 minutes, then season to taste.

To make the pesto, pound the garlic with the nuts in a pestle and mortar (alternatively whizz in a food processor). Add the basil leaves by small handfuls; gradually add the oil at the same time, continuing to pound and grind in a mortar. When all the leaves are ground to a somewhat smooth texture, stir in the remaining oil and the cheese, and season to taste. Serve bowls of soup with pesto to swirl on the top.

Warm salads

Warm vegetable salad

Slow cooked tomatoes are simply delicious for a change. However, if you are not keen on keeping the oven on for 4–5 hours, use sun-blush tomatoes instead of oven dried.

Serves: 4
Preparation time: 20 minutes
Cooking time: 4–5 hours

6 Roma tomatoes, halved
1 red pepper
1 yellow pepper
1 aubergine
2 courgettes
1 red onion, peeled
6 field mushrooms
4 baby yellow squash
vegetable oil
bag of baby lettuce leaves

for the dressing:
1 tbsp virgin olive oil
1 tbsp balsamic vinegar
1 clove garlic, peeled and finely chopped
1 tsp each of honey, wholegrain mustard, lemon juice
sea salt flakes, freshly ground black pepper

Preheat the oven to 110°C/225°F/gas mark ¼. Put the halved tomatoes on to a flat baking sheet and roast for 4–5 hours, or until semi dried. Heat a grill to high and cook the peppers, skin side up, until blistered and black all over. Put the peppers into a plastic bag (the steam helps to loosen the skins), leave to cool, then peel. Slice the pepper flesh into thin strips. Cut the aubergine, courgette and onion into thick slices, brush with oil and griddle for a couple of minutes until they are slightly soft and beginning to char in places. Put all of the salad ingredients in a bowl. Mix together the dressing ingredients and season well. Drizzle the dressing over the vegetables, add the lettuce leaves, toss together and serve.

Fresh tuna Niçoise

Prepare the salad in advance and cook the tuna on a griddle or, if you are lucky with the weather, a barbeque. It only takes minutes to sear the fish on the outside, keeping it raw in the middle.

Serves: 6
Preparation time: 15 minutes
Cooking time: 15–20 minutes

150 g/5 oz new potatoes, scrubbed
6 eggs
150 g/5 oz runner beans, trimmed
6 skinless tuna steaks (or use canned tuna, if fresh is not available)
125 g/4 oz fresh mixed baby salad leaves
225 g/8 oz ripe baby tomatoes, halved
150 g/5 oz black olives
6 spring onions, finely sliced
10 anchovy fillets
lots of lemon and lime wedges, to serve

for the dressing:
100 ml/3 fl oz olive oil
juice of 1 lime and 1 lemon
1 clove garlic, peeled and finely chopped
fresh flat leaf parsley, roughly chopped

Bring a pan of water to the boil, add the potatoes and boil for 10–12 minutes, or until soft. Drain and halve. Put the eggs into a small saucepan, cover with water, and quickly bring up to the boil. Reduce the heat to a simmer and cook the eggs for 3 minutes (cooked this way they will have slightly runny yolks), plunge straight into cold water, crack the shells and peel. Put the beans into a bowl and cover with boiling water. Leave for a couple of seconds to blanch, then refresh in cold water. Preheat a griddle and cook the tuna – as for 1 minute each side for rare, 2 minutes for medium and 3 for well done. Cut each tuna steak in half. Put the salad leaves into a big serving dish and top with the potatoes, beans, tomatoes, olives, onions and anchovies. Put the oil, juice of lemon and lime and seasoning into a bowl and mix well. Drizzle half of the dressing over the salad and toss everything together, including the egg. Serve the salad and top each with a couple of pieces of tuna, drizzle over the remaining dressing (to taste) and enjoy.

Top tips:

If frozen, do not thaw fish by soaking in water as this will destroy the texture and reduce the nutrient content. Tuna is a natural oil-rich fish and therefore contains the essential fatty acid omega 3, which helps to lower blood cholesterol.

If you are buying canned tuna, buy the water-based variety. Omega 3 is absorbed into the oil of the oil-packed variety, which is then drained off.

Anchovies can be very salty so either rinse in water, pat dry or soak in milk for 20 minutes then pat dry.

Bacon and glazed chicken livers

For those of you who are not too keen on livers, this is a delicious way to enjoy them.

Serves: 4
Preparation time: 15 minutes
Cooking time: 10 minutes

8 rashers back bacon
1 red onion, peeled and sliced into thin wedges
1 tbsp olive oil
25 g/1 oz butter
450 g/1 lb chicken livers, trimmed
1½ tbsp balsamic vinegar
handful fresh chives, chopped
300 g/11 oz salad leaves (mixed leaves)
sea salt flakes, freshly ground black pepper
chunks of crusty bread, to serve

Preheat the grill to high and cook the bacon until crispy, then keep warm. Heat the oil, fry the onion until golden brown, remove from the pan and put into a large bowl. Add the butter to the pan and sear the chicken livers until golden, but still soft inside (you may need to do this in batches). Add to the onions and keep warm. Deglaze the pan with balsamic vinegar. Cut the bacon into little strips and add to the liver with the chives and salad leaves. Drizzle over the juices from the pan and toss everything together. Season and serve with crusty bread.

Couscous with grilled tomatoes and red onions

I have a real passion for couscous, one of the truly great dishes of Morocco, Tunisia and Algeria. The small creamy coloured grains are made from strong or hard wheat, moistened with water, coated with a fine flour, then formed into tiny pellets. Like many other staple carbohydrates, couscous relies on the ingredients that you add to it for flavour and contrasting texture. This salad is a good example of just that. The couscous is packed with flavour and is simply delicious as the warm tomato juice soaks into the little pellets.

Serves: 4
Preparation time: 20 minutes (plus 30 minutes soaking time)
Cooking time: 10–15 minutes

350 g/12 oz couscous
350 ml/12 fl oz hot vegetable stock or water
sea salt flakes, freshly ground black pepper
450 g/1 lb big juicy tomatoes
2 tbsp olive oil
3 cloves garlic, peeled and chopped
handful black olives, stoned
handful fresh basil leaves, torn
large handful fresh flat leaf parsley, roughly chopped
juice of ½ lemon

for the dressing:
4 tbsp olive oil
2 red onions, peeled and thinly sliced
1 tbsp balsamic vinegar
sea salt flakes, freshly ground black pepper

Put the couscous into an ovenproof dish and pour over the hot vegetable stock (or water), then season. Cover and leave for 20 minutes in a warm place. Cut the tomatoes into thick slices. Heat half of the oil in a frying pan and fry the garlic for a couple of minutes, without browning. Add half of the tomato slices and cook until slightly golden on both sides, then put onto a plate. Add the other tablespoon of olive oil, repeat with the rest of the tomatoes and keep warm.

For the dressing; heat the olive oil in a pan, add the onion and cook until soft. Turn off the heat, add the vinegar and season. Fluff up the couscous with a fork, add the olives and herbs and season to taste with lemon juice. Mix everything together and divide between four serving plates. Top each with the hot garlicky tomatoes. Spoon over the onions and drizzle over the dressing.

Top tips:

To store parsley, cut off the bottom of the parsley roots, place the stems in cold water, and cover with a plastic bag.

To stone olives, bash with a flat object (such as a rolling pin or small bowl) and remove stone.

Roasted asparagus with a lime vinaigrette

Serve this with fresh bread or indulge yourself and eat as a mid-afternoon snack.

Serves: 4
Preparation time: 15 minutes (plus 10 minutes standing time)
Cooking time: 15 minutes

450 g/1 lb asparagus
4 tbsp extra virgin olive oil
sea salt flakes, freshly ground black pepper
1 shallot
1 tbsp red wine vinegar
1 lime or lemon, thinly sliced

Preheat the oven to 200°C/400°F/gas mark 6. Wash the asparagus and trim the thick ends. Put the asparagus into a roasting tin, in a single layer, and drizzle with half of the oil. Roll the spears to coat with oil, and season. Cook at the top of the oven for 15 minutes, until soft when pierced with a knife. Make the vinaigrette; put the shallot, vinegar and lime or lemon slices into a bowl, toss everything together and leave for 10 minutes. Add the rest of the oil to the vinegar and season to taste. Arrange the asparagus on serving plates and drizzle with vinaigrette. Serve at room temperature.

Top tips:

Asparagus is a good cleanser and diuretic.

New potato salad

Instead of the traditional salad of potatoes tossed in a mayonnaise-based creamy dressing, this salad has attitude with the sharp lemon juice and peppery watercress. This recipe needs new potatoes, which are harvested when the tubers are still immature and the skins have not quite set, hence they can be rubbed off relatively easily. New potatoes do not keep that well, so try to eat them as quickly as possible after purchase.

Serves: 4
Preparation time: 15 minutes
Cooking time: 10–12 minutes

550 g/1¼ lb new potatoes
1½ tbsp lemon juice
3 tbsp extra virgin olive oil
sea salt flakes, freshly ground black pepper
handful of each flat-leaf parsley and basil leaves, chopped
2 carrots, trimmed
2 sticks celery
large handful fresh watercress, roughly chopped
2 red pepper, seeded and finely sliced

Bring a pan of water to the boil, add the potatoes and cook for 10–12 minutes, until tender when pierced with a knife. Drain and cut in half. Whisk the lemon juice and oil together, season well. Pour the dressing over the warm potatoes (they will absorb the flavour from the dressing into their flesh). Add the parsley and basil, mix everything together and leave to stand for 10 minutes. Thinly slice the carrots and celery. Add to the potatoes with the watercress and red pepper. Mix everything together, season to taste and serve.

Cold salads

Cannellini beans with tomatoes and basil

The cannellini bean is starchy and versatile. I often serve this lunch with sour dough and a big bowl of black olives.

Serves: 4
Preparation time: 20 minutes
Cooking time: 20–25 minutes

275 g/10 oz dried cannellini beans, soaked overnight
1 bay leaf
sprigs of fresh marjoram, thyme and sage
2 tbsp red wine vinegar
zest of 2 lemons
2 garlic cloves, peeled and finely chopped
sea salt flakes, freshly ground black pepper
extra virgin olive oil
225 g/8 oz tomatoes
¼ red onion, peeled
large handful (about 10 g/ ½ oz) fresh basil leaves, torn
champagne vinegar, to taste
sour dough and black olives, to serve

Drain and rinse the beans and place them in a large saucepan. Cover generously with cold water, then add the bay leaf and herb sprigs. Bring to the boil, then reduce the heat and cook at a gentle boil until tender, for about 20–25 minutes. Taste the beans to be sure that they're cooked through. If the skins are still tough, cook them a little longer until they loosen and begin to open. Combine the red wine vinegar, lemon zest, garlic, salt and pepper in a bowl and whisk in the oil. Core and seed the tomatoes, then cut into the large pieces. Drain the cooked beans and toss them immediately with vinaigrette. The hot beans will soak up all the good flavours. Cool, then add the tomatoes, onion and basil. Season to taste and add champagne vinegar if needed.

Top tips:

Cannellini beans, as with other dried beans, should be soaked overnight and then cooked before use. They should be rinsed in a sieve to remove any floury matter before cooking as this will reduce the scum.

The longer you keep dried pulses, the harder they become and therefore the longer they take to cook.

Peas, beans and lentils are valuable sources of protein, iron, calcium, zinc, magnesium and B vitamins. They also contain a special kind of dietary fibre, which can help to regulate the control of glucose in the body.

Sandwiches

Chicken with sun-dried tomatoes and avocado

Selection of olives and nuts

Chocolate and berry cake

Tomato and watercress salad with hazelnut dressing

I love watercress because of its fabulous peppery flavour and crunchy texture. It is also very versatile because it is in season the whole year around. Hampshire is the area famous for its watercress, around the valleys that have chalk springs.

Serves: 4
Preparation time: 10 minutes

2 tsp balsamic vinegar
2 tsp hazelnut oil
2 tsp dry white wine
1 tsp Dijon mustard
250 g/9 oz watercress
¼ red onion, peeled and finely chopped
8 ripe tomatoes
sea salt flakes, freshly ground black pepper

Put the vinegar, oil, wine and mustard into a small bowl and whisk together, then season to taste. Wash the watercress and scatter over a small platter. Add the onion to the vinaigrette. Chop the tomatoes into thin slices and scatter over the watercress. Drizzle the vinaigrette over the salad, season well and serve.

Top tips:

Watercress leaves are packed with the vitamins C and B and many minerals including sulphur, potassium, calcium and phosphorous. I believe watercress is underused and underrated in our cooking today.

As with other cold dishes, watercress adds colour, texture and a peppery kick to this crispy salad. It is also great added to hot dishes, especially stir-fries. Add just before the end of cooking so that the pretty green leaves are given just enough time to wilt.

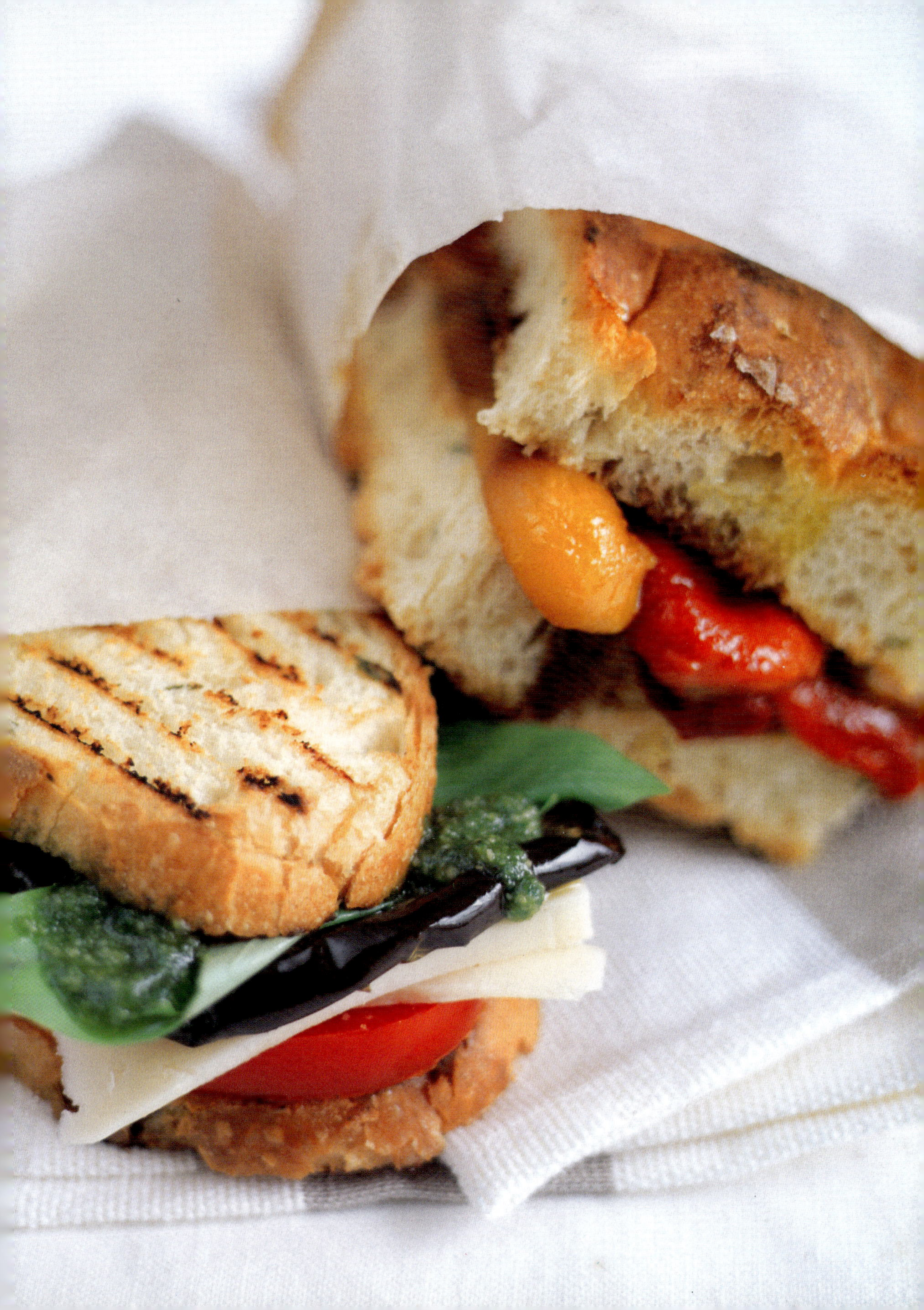

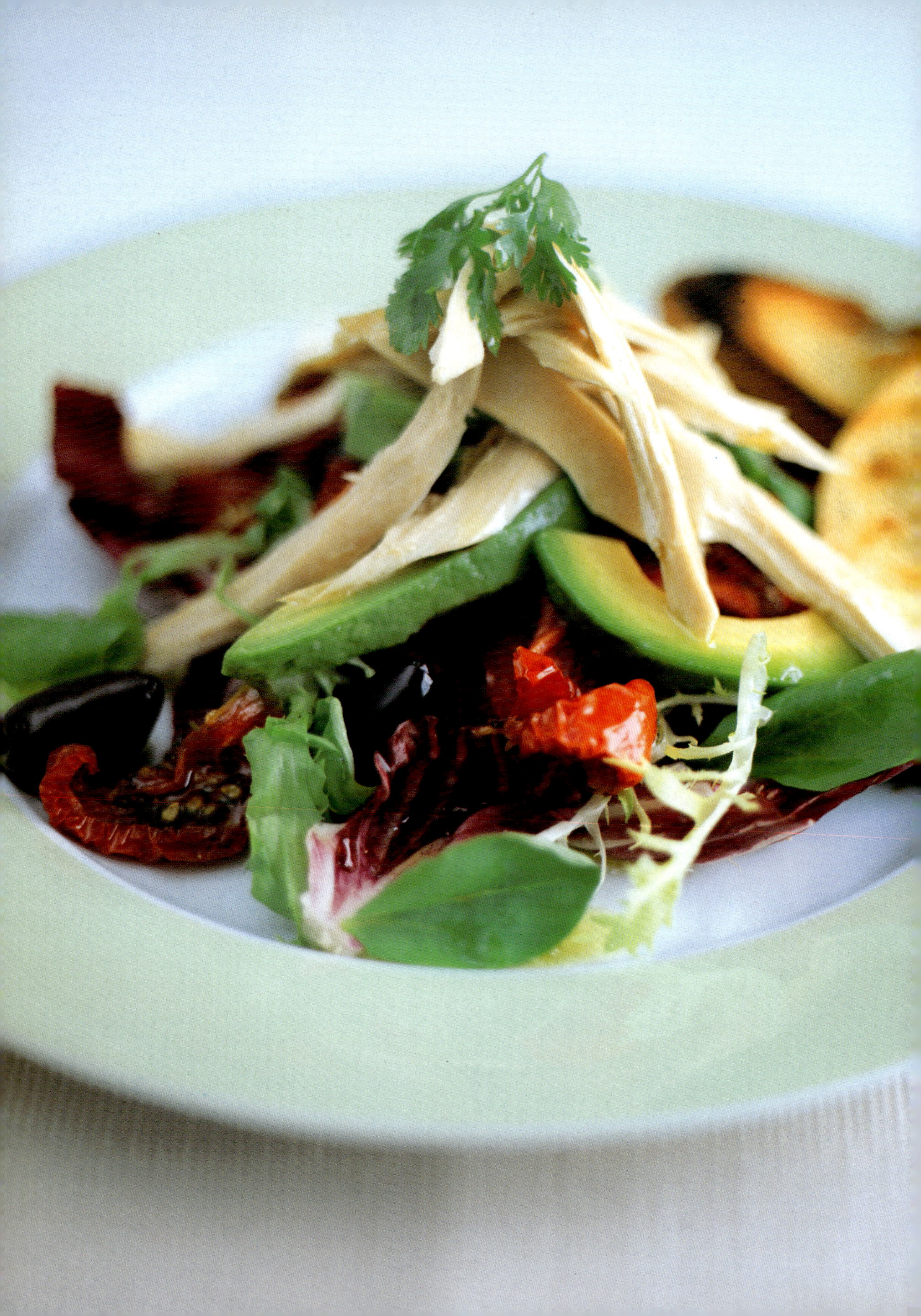

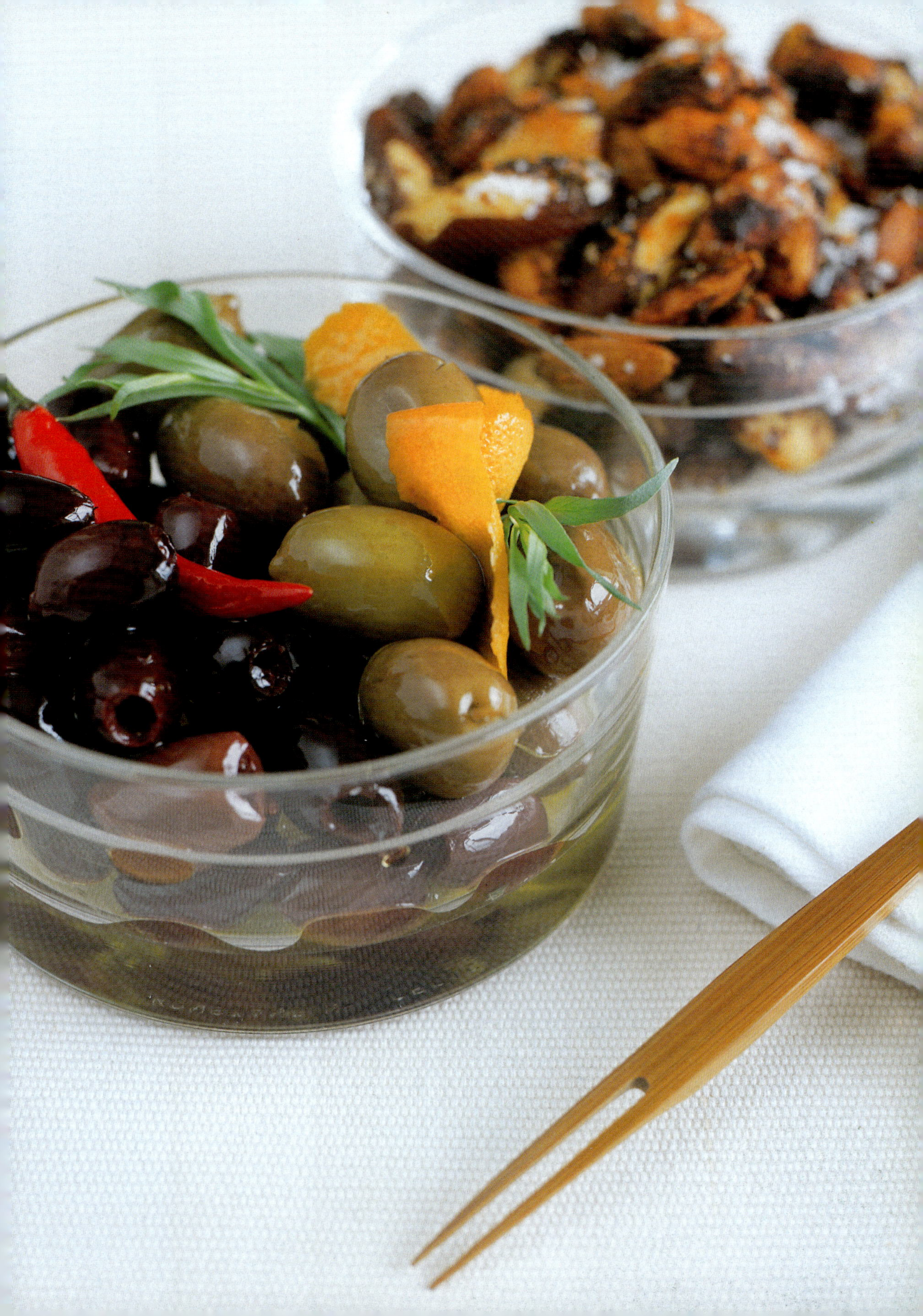

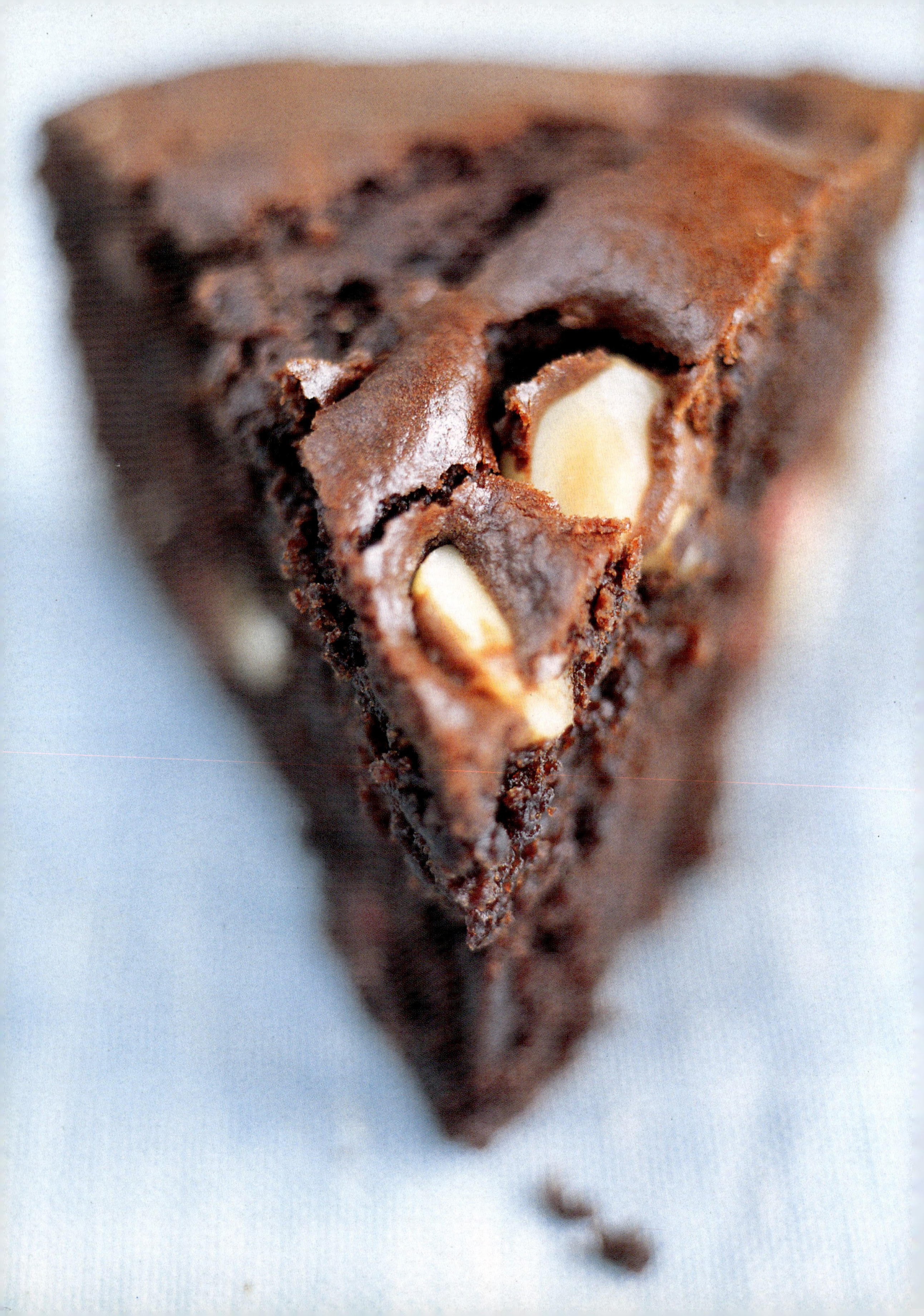

Watercress, orange and fennel

Watercress, a semi-aquatic herb, grows wild in British lowlands, either in ditches or streams, or anywhere near running water. I love its wild appearance, which makes it seem so uncontrollable and full of life. For a very quick snack, cut a ciabatta loaf in half, brush the insides with a little oil and pack the bread with watercress (I have been known to use 150 g/5 oz in one loaf). Season the watercress and cut the loaf into two or three sandwiches (the layers of watercress look amazing) then eat.

This is delicious as a lunch, especially served with Creamy smoked mackerel (see page 110). Alternatively, it makes a great refreshing starter.

Serves: 4
Preparation time: 20 minutes

2 big juicy oranges
1 bulb fennel, trimmed
75 g/3 oz watercress
sea salt flakes, freshly ground black pepper

for the dressing:
2 tbsp orange juice
1 tsp honey
2 tbsp extra virgin olive oil

Cut the top and bottom off the oranges. Peel the oranges; work your way around the oranges with a sharp knife, removing the skin and white pith. Cut out each segment from the fruit and put into a bowl (catch any juice as you work for the dressing). Cut the fennel into quarters, cut out the hard core and then cut each quarter into long thin slices. Put the fennel into a bowl. Add the watercress and orange to the fennel, mix together and season to taste. Put the dressing ingredients into a jar and shake together. Drizzle the dressing over the salad, leave for 5 minutes, then serve.

Baby spinach with crispy bacon and soft creamy eggs

Different varieties of spinach are available in spring, summer and autumn. I prefer the young leaves for salads like these and the larger leaves slightly wilted in stir-fries or other dishes.

Serves: 4
Preparation time: 15 minutes
Cooking time: 20 minutes

1 small French baguette
virgin olive oil, to drizzle
4 large free-range eggs
8 rashers back bacon
225 g/8 oz young leaf spinach

for the lemon dressing:
2 tbsp extra virgin olive oil
juice of ½ lemon
sea salt flakes, freshly ground black pepper

Preheat the oven to 220°C/425°F/gas mark 7. Cut the bread into very thin diagonal slices, cut each slice in half, put on to a baking tray and drizzle with oil. Bake for 10 minutes, turning every now and then (keep an eye on the bread, it may catch quite quickly). Bring a pan of water to the boil, add the eggs and boil for 6 minutes, then drain and plunge into cold water. Grill the bacon until crispy and cut into thin strips. Put the bacon and croûtons into a bowl, add the spinach and mix together. Put the dressing ingredients into a jar and shake together. Divide the salads between four serving plates, and top each with wedges of egg (the yolk should be slightly runny in the centre). Drizzle over the dressing and serve.

Tomatoes with fresh basil and Parmesan

This makes a very quick, light lunch. Serve with fresh bread to add carbohydrate.

Serves: 4
Preparation time: 10 minutes

6 tomatoes
sea salt flakes, freshly ground black pepper
1 clove garlic, peeled and finely chopped
handful fresh basil leaves, shredded
3 tbsp extra virgin olive oil
75 g/3 oz Parmesan cheese shavings
handful basil leaves, to garnish

Cut the tomatoes into slices, wedges or halves, depending on their size, arrange on a platter and season well. Mix the garlic, shredded basil leaves and oil together and drizzle over the tomatoes. Scatter over the Parmesan shavings and a few more fresh basil leaves, then serve.

Spinach with satsumas and a ginger vinaigrette

This is refreshing, easy to prepare and the dressing of ginger and sesame is a marriage made in heaven.

Serves: 4
Preparation time: 15 minutes

2 handfuls frisée or chicory
450 g/1 lb young leaf spinach
½ red onion, peeled and finely chopped
3 satsumas (or 2 blood oranges)
handful sesame seeds, toasted

for the ginger and sesame vinaigrette:
2 tbsp satsuma juice (or blood orange juice)
2.5 cm/1 inch piece fresh root ginger, peeled and grated
2½ tbsp rice wine vinegar
2 tbsp light olive oil
1 tbsp sesame oil
1 tsp soy sauce
pinch salt
1 tsp satsuma zest (or blood orange zest)

Cut off the stem end of the frisée and discard the tough outer leaves. Put the pale green inner leaves into a colander with the spinach, wash and dry. Peel and section the satsumas, removing any seeds. Make the vinaigrette; put everything, except the zest, in a food processor and blend. Whisk in the zest. Combine the greens, satsumas and onion in a bowl. Toss with the vinaigrette and sprinkle with sesame seeds.

Top tip:

Citrus juices help to clean the digestive system. Cells, capillaries, heart and lungs all benefit from our citric friends and they also help to promote healthy skin.

Baby spinach with mushrooms, pine nuts and blue cheese

The mushrooms, pine nuts and cheese make a wonderful combination.

Serves: 4
Preparation time: 20 minutes
Cooking time: 15 minutes

25 g/1 oz pine nuts
400 g/14 oz mixed mushrooms, such as oyster or button mushrooms
1 tbsp olive oil
100 g/3½ oz blue cheese, crumbled (Danish Blue, Roquefort or Dolcelatte)
225 g/8 oz young leaf spinach leaves, washed and large stalks removed

for the dressing:
3 tbsp extra virgin olive oil
1 tbsp balsamic vinegar
1 clove garlic, peeled and finely chopped
sea salt flakes, freshly ground black pepper

Dry fry the pine nuts until golden, this will take approximately 3 minutes. Cut the big mushrooms into thick slices (leaving the small mushrooms whole). Heat the oil in a large frying pan, add the mushrooms and cook over a high heat for 4–5 minutes until golden. Add the cheese to the pan and warm through until the cheese just starts to melt. Divide the spinach leaves between four plates, then top with the cheese and mushroom mixture. In a separate bowl or screw-top jar, mix together the dressing ingredients and drizzle over the salads. You may need more balsamic vinegar, just add to taste.

Top tips:

Spinach is full of dark green chlorophyll and rich in minerals, especially iron.

Garlic is the king of all healing plants. No other plant has enjoyed such a reputation in so many different countries and civilisations for helping such a wide range of ailments, or been the subject of such intensive modern research.

Tomato salad with cucumbers, feta cheese, oregano and mint

All you need to go with salads like these is a little sun and a table in the garden.

Serves: 4
Preparation time: 25 minutes

150 g/5 oz mixed salad leaves
450 g/1 lb vine-ripened tomatoes
½ small cucumber
125 g/4 oz feta, crumbled
handful each fresh oregano and mint, roughly chopped

for the lemon vinaigrette:
zest of ½ lemon
2 tbsp fresh lemon juice
½ tbsp champagne vinegar
50 ml/2 fl oz extra virgin olive oil
sea salt flakes, freshly ground black pepper

Wash and dry the leaves. Core the tomatoes and slice into thick rounds or wedges. Peel and seed the cucumber and slice 5 mm/¼ inch thick on a diagonal. Add the tomatoes, cucumber and feta to the leaves. Make the vinaigrette; put everything in a small bowl and whisk. Drizzle the vinaigrette over the salad, scatter over the herbs, season to taste with salt and lots of freshly ground black pepper and serve.

Soft garlicky peppers

The flavours in this salad improve over time. This is delicious served with grilled fish or chicken.

Serves: 4
Preparation time: 20 minutes (plus 1 hour minimum marinating time)
Cooking time: 15 minutes

3 ripe red peppers
2 yellow peppers
3 tbsp extra virgin olive oil
1 small garlic, peeled and crushed
handful fresh coriander, roughly chopped
zest of 1 lemon
sea salt flakes, freshly ground black pepper
1 tbsp white wine vinegar
handful fresh coriander leaves, roughly chopped, to garnish

Put the peppers under a hot grill and cook until black all over (approximately 10–15 minutes). Put the peppers straight into a plastic bag and leave for 5 minutes: the steam helps to release the skins. Peel, then cut the flesh into strips and put straight into a serving bowl. In a separate bowl, mix together the oil, garlic, coriander and lemon zest, then season to taste. Pour the dressing over the peppers and leave to marinate for several hours. Take the dish out of the fridge at least 20 minutes before serving, drizzle over the vinegar, scatter over fresh coriander leaves and serve.

Pepper salad

This makes a perfect lunch served with some fresh crusty ciabatta to mop up the juices. This salad keeps well and its flavours actually improve with time.

Serves: 4
Preparation time: 15 minutes
Cooking time: 20 minutes

8 long red peppers
100 g/3½ oz Mahon or other cheese
75 g/3 oz Spanish olives
bunch fresh flat leaf parsley, roughly chopped
1–2 tbsp extra virgin olive oil
sea salt flakes, freshly ground black pepper
ciabatta or crusty bread, to serve

Preheat the grill to high, cut the peppers in half lengthways and grill skin side up until black all over (this will take approximately 10 minutes). Put the peppers straight into a bowl, cover with cling film and leave for 5 minutes. Peel the peppers and put into a salad bowl. Slice the cheese as finely as possible, add to the peppers. Bash the olives with a flat bowl and remove the stones. Add the olives to the peppers with the parsley, drizzle with oil and season. Mix everything together and serve with crusty bread.

Pear, fennel and walnut salad

Eat freshly shelled nuts whenever possible as nuts have a high fat content and can go rancid quite quickly once shelled.

Serves: 4
Preparation time: 20 minutes

4 firm, ripe pears
juice of 1 lemon
3 baby fennel bulbs, trimmed
3 tbsp walnut pieces
2 radicchio hearts
bunch fresh rocket
1–2 tbsp walnut oil, to taste
sea salt flakes, freshly ground black pepper

Peel, core and slice the pears lengthways. Put into a serving bowl, add the lemon juice and toss to coat. Slice the fennel into thin strips and add to the pears. Dry fry the walnut pieces for a few seconds, until slightly golden (this helps to bring out their flavour). Tear the radicchio leaves into smaller pieces, add to the pears with the fresh rocket and toasted walnuts. Mix everything together, drizzle over the walnut oil, season to taste and serve.

Top tips:

It has been said that walnuts are the most nutritious of all the nuts. Pears are said have roughly the same amount of fibre as a cup and a half of brown rice and more than a serving of muesli. Slice pears and serve with smoked mackerel for a very quick lunch.

Watercress with red chilli and basil

We take it for granted that garlic is available all year round, which sadly means that many people miss out on the experience of tasting the new season garlic, which appears in the middle of the summer. Make a point of keeping an eye out for the fresh, soft, purple bulbs in summer and use generously in your cooking while it is in plentiful supply.

Serves: 4
Preparation time: 10 minutes

juice of ½ lemon
1 red chilli, seeded and sliced
2 tsp sugar
3 tbsp olive oil
1 tsp balsamic vinegar
1 clove garlic, peeled and finely sliced
2 tbsp white wine
basil leaves, roughly torn
sea salt flakes, freshly ground black pepper
2 large bunches watercress

Put all of the ingredients, except the watercress, into a jar and shake well. Put the watercress into a bowl and drizzle the dressing over the top. Toss to mix everything together, season to taste and serve.

Chickpeas and sun-blush tomatoes with fresh herb dressing

I have used dried chickpeas in this salad to encourage the flavours from the dressing to soak into the beans. However, to save time, you could use canned.

Serves: 4
Preparation time: 20 minutes (plus 1 hour marinating time)
Cooking time: 50–60 minutes

275 g/10 oz dried chickpeas, soaked overnight
1 bay leaf
1 fresh sage leaf
2 fresh marjoram sprigs
50 ml/2 fl oz red wine vinegar
1 garlic clove, peeled and finely chopped
sea salt flakes, freshly ground black pepper
2 tbsp extra virgin olive oil
½ small red onion, peeled and diced
2 sun-blush tomatoes, roughly chopped
handful fresh parsley, roughly chopped
crispy croûtons, to serve

Drain and rinse the chickpeas. Put them into large saucepan, cover with water, add the bay leaf and herbs and bring to the boil. Boil gently for 20–30 minutes, until the beans are tender. Combine the red wine vinegar, garlic, salt and pepper. Gradually whisk in the oil. Drain the beans, add the vinaigrette, onion and sun-blush tomatoes and marinate for an hour. Add the parsley and season to taste. Serve sprinked with crispy croûtons.

Carrot with nuts and raisins in a tangy orange dressing

Carrots first appear in the gardens in late spring, although, like many vegetables, we see them all year round in the shops. Toasting the nuts really brings out their flavour.

Serves: 4
Preparation time: 10 minutes (plus 20 minutes marinating time)

50 g/2 oz hazelnuts, chopped
400 g/14 oz carrots
75 g/3 oz raisins
125 g/4 oz black olives, stoned
2–3 tbsp sesame seeds

for the dressing:
3 tbsp extra virgin olive oil
1 tbsp fresh orange juice
2 tbsp fresh coriander, roughly chopped
zest and juice of ½ lemon
sea salt flakes, freshly ground black pepper

Dry fry the hazelnuts until golden. Grate the carrots and put into a bowl. Add the raisins, hazelnuts and olives and mix together. Put all of the dressing ingredients into a bowl, mix well and drizzle over the salad. Season to taste. Leave to stand at room temperature for at least 20 minutes. Toast the sesame seeds in a dry frying pan until golden and scatter over the salad.

Broad bean salad with ham or cheese

From June to September we can buy and enjoy fresh broad beans. Shelling the beans may seem like a lot of effort, but trust me, it's worth it. This recipe is particularly scrummy as the warm beans absorb the flavours from the dressing.

Serves: 4
Preparation time: 20 minutes
Cooking time: 15–20 minutes

700 g/1½ lb shelled broad beans
125 g/4 oz ham or cheese, thinly sliced

for the vinaigrette:
juice of 1 lemon
2–3 tbsp extra virgin olive oil
sea salt flakes, freshly ground black pepper
2 tbsp fresh mint, roughly chopped

Bring a pan of water to the boil, add the beans and cook until just tender, drain and put into a bowl. Put the vinaigrette ingredients into a screw-top jar and shake well. Pour the vinaigrette over the warm beans and leave to cool. Cut the ham or cheese into thin slices, then add to the beans with the mint. Toss everything together and serve.

Top tip:

Broad beans are sometimes known as fava beans.

Wild rice salad with tangerines and pine nuts

Champagne vinegar accents citric juices.

Serves: 4
Preparation time: 15–20 minutes
Cooking time: 25 minutes

200 g/7 oz wild and basmati rice
150 ml/5 fl oz fresh tangerine juice (juice of approx 4 tangerines)
85 g/3½ oz dried currants or cranberries (or a mixture of the two)
3 tangerines
1 tbsp champagne vinegar
2 tbsp light olive oil
2 tbsp pine nuts, toasted
sea salt flakes, freshly ground black pepper

Bring a large pan of water to the boil, stir in the rice and cook for about 20 minutes, then drain. Put the tangerine juice in a small saucepan and bring slowly up to the boil. Remove from the heat, add the currants or cranberries and leave for a few minutes until plump (about 3 minutes). Peel and segment the tangerines, then add to the rice. Add the champagne vinegar and olive oil to the currants, mix together and pour half over the rice. Leave to cool. Add the toasted pine nuts and season to taste. Serve with the rest of the currant mixture.

Lentils with herbs and balsamic vinegar

Serve this with some pitta and houmous and you have a satisfying lunch.

Serves: 4
Preparation time: 15 minutes

2 x 400 g cans Puy or green lentils, drained and rinsed
juice of 1 lemon
1 tbsp balsamic vinegar
½ red onion, peeled and chopped
2 tbsp fresh thyme leaves, roughly chopped
sea salt flakes, freshly ground black pepper
5 ripe vine tomatoes

Put the lentils into a bowl. Add the lemon juice, balsamic vinegar, red onion and thyme, season well and mix together. Chop the tomatoes, seed, cut the flesh into little pieces, and add to the lentils.

Top tip:

Lentils provide large amounts of dietary fibre, protein, complex carbohydrate and an impressive amount of iron, thiamine, niacin, phosphorous and potassium.

Chicken with avocado

Another protein-packed lunch with maximum flavour, from a chef friend, Clint

Serves: 4
Preparation time: 15 minutes
Cooking time: 5 minutes

1 large radicchio
6 medium endive
200 g/7 oz lamb's lettuce
1 red pepper, cut in half and seeded
2 tbsp olive oil and 100 ml/3 fl oz extra virgin olive oil
1 clove garlic, peeled and finely crushed
1 small baguette, thinly sliced
25 ml/1 fl oz balsamic vinegar
1 tbsp golden caster sugar
sea salt flakes, freshly ground black pepper
4 pieces organic chicken, cooked
2 ripe avocados
200 g/7 oz sun-dried tomatoes, roughly chopped
24 black olives (Kalamata), stoned
fresh coriander or chervil, roughly chopped

Preheat a grill to medium. Tear the radicchio, break up the endive and wash both of them with the lamb's lettuce. Leave to drain. Thinly slice the red pepper and put into a bowl of iced water. Mix together 2 tablespoons of the oil with the garlic. Brush the baguette with the garlic oil and toast evenly on both sides. Put the lettuces into a bowl. Make the dressing; mix together the remaining oil, vinegar and sugar and season to taste. Drizzle over the lettuce and toss everything together. Arrange the lettuce on four plates and put the bruschetta on the side. Shred the chicken into thin strips. Stone, peel and cut the avocado flesh into cubes. Put the chicken, avocado, tomatoes and olives into a bowl and mix everything together. Pile this mixture into the middle of each plate. Finish with the pepper strips and scatter over the chopped herbs.

Beef with rocket and balsamic vinegar

This is a very simple salad, but a great combination of ingredients. If you can get hold of 'wild' rocket, use it.

Serves: 4
Preparation time: 5 minutes

8 ripe and juicy tomatoes
8 slices of cooked beef
sea salt flakes, freshly ground black pepper
4 tsp balsamic vinegar, to taste
50 g/2oz baby (or wild) rocket
handful of Parmesan cheese shavings

Slice the tomatoes and divide between four plates. Top with the beef and season with salt and pepper, and drizzle each with balsamic vinegar. Top with fresh rocket and Parmesan shavings, and serve.

Homemade sea salt and rosemary flat breads

These are great served with dips (see pages xxx) and fresh vegetables. It is surprising how quickly they cook, you just need to be in a patient mood to give the dough time to rise. I always enjoy making bread, I find kneading the dough very therapeutic.

Makes: about 20
Preparation time: 30 minutes (plus 3½ hours rising time)
Cooking time: about 20 minutes

1 tsp active dry yeast
600 ml/1 pint warm water
500 g/1 lb 2 oz strong wholemeal flour
2 tsp sea salt flakes
1 tbsp extra virgin olive oil
360 g/12½ oz–425 g/15 oz plain flour

for the topping:
extra virgin olive oil
sea salt flakes
fresh sprigs rosemary and other herbs

Dissolve the yeast in the water. Put the flour in a bowl, make a well in the middle, add the yeast mixture and mix until well combined. Cover with cling film and leave to stand in a warm place for 1 hour 30 minutes or until doubled in size. Mix in the sea salt and oil. Gradually add the plain flour (the mixture will be sticky at first) and knead the dough as you add the flour, until you have a smooth dough. Knead for 8 minutes. Cover the dough with cling film and leave for about 2 hours, until double in size. Divide the dough into about 16 pieces and roll each piece into a ball. Roll out the balls on a lightly floured surface until they are 4 mm/¼ inch thick. Brush one side of the dough with oil, scatter over the sea salt flakes and stick the rosemary sprigs into the dough. Leave the dough to rise for 10 minutes. Cook the flat breads under a preheated grill or on a griddle pan for 1–2 minutes on each side or until they are puffed and golden.

Top tip:

Rosemary aids the digestion of fat and stimulates the circulation. It is a good 'pick-me-up' and it can help ease aching joints. Rosemary stems stripped of their lower leaves act as good skewers for grilling meat or vegetables. Scatter a few rosemary sprigs over vegetables, lamb, fowl and strong-flavoured fish such as tuna and swordfish during cooking.

Couscous with fruits and spices

Couscous is like pasta, it relies on the ingredients that you add to it for flavour. Use a good liquid (or combination of liquids, as in this recipe) to soak into the couscous, rather than simply using water.

Serves: 4
Preparation time: 20 minutes
Cooking time: 5 minutes

200 g/7 oz couscous
4 fl oz/125 ml water
125 ml/4 fl oz/fresh orange juice
2 tbsp light olive oil
2 tbsp champagne vinegar
100 g/3½ oz dried apricots, roughly chopped (preferably organic without sulphur)
2 tbsp of each currants and raisins
2.5 cm/1 inch fresh ginger, peeled and grated
sea salt flakes, freshly ground black pepper
½ tsp of each paprika and cinnamon
¼ red onion, peeled and finely diced
3 tbsp pine nuts, toasted
fresh coriander, roughly chopped (optional)

Put the couscous into a bowl, then put the water, orange juice, olive oil and vinegar in a small saucepan. Bring the liquid just up to the boil, add the fruit, ginger, pinch of salt and spices, and pour over the couscous. Cover and leave in a warm place for at least 20 minutes. Fluff the couscous with a fork, add the onion, pine nuts and coriander (if using). Season to taste and serve.

Tomato puff with pesto and olives

Serves: 4
Preparation time: 15 minutes
Cooking time: 20 minutes

4 pastry circles
4 tbsp pesto (see page 85, or buy pesto from a deli)
5 ripe tomatoes
150 g/5 oz black olives, stoned
fresh basil leaves, to serve

Cook the pastry in the same way as above. Turn over and cover with the pesto, sliced tomatoes and olives. Return to the oven for 5 minutes to heat through. Scatter over the basil leaves and serve.

Vegetarian sushi

You need half an hour to prepare the Japanese rice, but apart from that this sushi is incredibly quick and very simple. I love little sushi rolls as a starter, it is not too filling if you only eat a few and more importantly it impresses every time.

Now, we are fortunate enough to be able to buy ingredients like konbu and nori seaweed, rice wine vinegar, pickled ginger and wasabi from some major supermarkets. The easiest way to buy wasabi (Japanese horseradish) is in a tube. Squeeze some into a little dish and use for dipping the sushi into, but go carefully, as it is incredibly hot.

Makes 30 pieces; serve about 5 pieces as a starter and 10 for a main course, per person
Preparation time: 20 minutes
Cooking time: 15 minutes (plus 15 minutes standing)

450 ml/ ¾ pint water
1 piece dashi konbu seaweed
225 g/8 oz Japanese rice for sushi
2 tbsp rice wine vinegar
1 tbsp caster sugar
pinch sea salt
1 avocado
½ cucumber
6 sheets nori seaweed
dark soy sauce, pickled ginger and wasabi, to serve

Alternative fillings – smoked salmon, mango strips, blanched asparagus, thin strips of omelette, strips of carrot, strips of radish

Put the water, dashi konbu and rice into a large pan. Bring to the boil, remove the dashi konbu, cover the rice and simmer for 10 minutes. Leave to stand (still covered) for 15 minutes, then transfer to a bowl. In a small bowl, mix together the vinegar, sugar and salt, stir into the rice and leave to cool.

Cut the cucumber in half lengthways and scrape out the seeds with a teaspoon. Stone and skin the avocado, then cut the cucumber and avocado flesh into long thin strips.

Place a nori sheet on a sushi mat and spoon rice over two thirds of it. Arrange a few strips of avocado and asparagus (or whichever combination you prefer) in the centre of the rice. Pick up the edge of the mat closest to you and roll the nori and filling away from you. Squash the roll to compress, then unroll the mat. Make up more rolls in the same way. Cut each roll into about 5 or 6 pieces. Serve with small dishes of soy sauce, pickled ginger and wasabi.

Jasmine rice pilaff with chunky tomato salsa

This is one of those lunches for when friends pop in. It is easy and quick to prepare.

Serves: 4
Preparation time: 20 minutes
Cooking time: 25–30 minutes

for the chunky tomato salsa:
450 g/1 lb ripe tomatoes
½ red onion, peeled and finely chopped
1 chilli, seeded and finely chopped
2 tbsp fresh coriander, roughly chopped
sea salt flakes, cayenne pepper

for the pilaff:
2 tbsp olive oil
2 onions, peeled and sliced
4 kaffir lime leaves
2 red chillies, seeded and finely sliced
300 g/11 oz jasmine rice
300 ml/11 fl oz of each vegetable stock and water
2 bunches fresh coriander, roughly chopped

Cut the tomatoes into small pieces and put into a bowl. Add the red onion, chilli and coriander. Season to taste with salt and cayenne pepper. Cover and put to one side to marinate. Add a drizzle of oil.

Meanwhile, make the pilaff; heat the oil in a heavy-based saucepan, add the onions and cook for 3 minutes, or until soft. Add the kaffir lime leaves and chillies and cook for a minute. Add rice, stock, water and half of the coriander to the pan, cover and simmer gently for 12 minutes. Remove the lid and cook for another 3 minutes (the rice should be cooked and the liquid absorbed). Add the rest of the coriander leaves and serve in warm bowls with the tomato salsa on the top.

Top tips:

Coriander leaves add a cooling quality to hot pungent foods.

Fresh coriander does not keep for a long time, so store in the same way as fresh parsley, but do not remove the roots or rinse the leaves until ready to use.

Tomato sauce for pasta

I developed this recipe one evening after a long photographic shoot. Annie, a close friend, came over for a chat and we were both so tired that we were not sure if we could muster up the energy to cook. Between us, with Annie chopping and me throwing things into a saucepan, we developed this very fast, very easy pasta sauce. It was such a hit with us and hubby (when the leftovers were reheated 2 hours later) that we decided it should definitely find its way into this book.

Serves: 3
Preparation time: 15 minutes
Cooking time: 10–15 minutes

2 tbsp olive oil
½ red onion, peeled and finely chopped
8–10 vine-ripened juicy red tomatoes
400 g can chopped tomatoes
2 tbsp tomato purée
1–2 tbsp good quality balsamic vinegar
2 tbsp really good juicy black olives, stoned
handful fresh coriander or parsley, roughly chopped
pasta of your choice, to serve
sea salt flakes, freshly ground black pepper
1–2 tbsp good homemade pesto

Heat the oil in a saucepan, add the onion and cook gently for 10 minutes, until soft. Roughly chop the fresh tomatoes and add to the saucepan with the canned tomatoes, tomato purée and balsamic vinegar. Simmer gently for 15 minutes. Add the olives, most of the herbs and cook for another 10 minutes, until it has reduced to a thick and intense tomato sauce. In the meantime, bring a pan of water to the boil, add the pasta and cook according to the packet instructions, then drain. Divide the pasta between four warm serving bowls. Season and add the pesto to the sauce, mix everything together and spoon on top of the pasta. Serve with plenty of fresh coriander or parsley scattered over.

Top tip:

Balsamic vinegar, which has a sweet sour flavour, is a speciality of Modena in Northern Italy. It is aged for ten, fifty or even a hundred years in oaked barrels. Some varieties are so rich and syrupy that they are sprinkled over fruit and served as a dessert.

Caramelised leek puff

The leek is one of the most desirable vegetables at a time when very little else is growing in the garden, they add colour, texture and flavour to our diet. Look out for leeks, depending on the variety, from between mid-autumn to late spring.

Serves: 4
Preparation time: 20 minutes
Cooking time: 25 minutes

5 leeks, trimmed
1 tbsp olive oil
2 onions, peeled and sliced
2 puff pastry sheets
75 g/3 oz Cheddar cheese, grated
handful fresh parsley, roughly chopped
sea salt flakes, freshly ground black pepper

Preheat the oven to 200°C/400°F/gas mark 6. Thinly slice the leeks. Heat the oil in a frying pan, add the leeks and onions, cover and sweat for 20 minutes. Meanwhile, cut four circles out of the pastry (use a saucer as a template) and score the edges with a sharp knife (this helps the pastry to rise). Rest the pastry on a baking sheet and bake for 15 minutes until golden and puffy. Turn the pastry circles over and cover with the leeks, then top with grated cheese. Scatter over the parsley and season well. Bake for another 5 minutes to heat through then serve.

Spaghetti with marinated tomatoes, fresh basil and garlic crumbs

Marinate the tomatoes for 30 minutes and the rest is very quick and simple.

Serves: 4
Preparation time: 20 minutes
Cooking time: 10–15 minutes

700 g/1½ lb vine-ripened tomatoes
50 ml/2 fl oz extra virgin olive oil
4 garlic cloves, peeled and finely chopped
handful fresh basil, roughly torn
sea salt flakes, freshly ground black pepper
225 g/8 oz spaghetti
50 g/2 oz breadcrumbs
fresh basil leaves, to serve

Chop the tomatoes into small chunks and put into a bowl. Add the oil, 3 of the chopped garlic cloves and basil, and season to taste. Leave to marinate for at least 30 minutes. Bring a large pan of water to the boil and cook the spaghetti according to the packet instructions, then drain. Put the breadcrumbs and remaining chopped garlic on to a baking tray, mix together and toast until golden. Mix the spaghetti with the tomato mixture and divide between four warm bowls. Scatter the garlic crumbs over the top, followed by a few fresh basil leaves and serve.

Pasta with lemon, rocket and chilli

This tastes fresh and is a wonderful way to eat an energy-packed lunch of carbohydrate and vitamins.

Serves: 4
Preparation time: 15 minutes
Cooking time: 10–15 minutes

700 g/1½ lb pasta shells
4 tbsp olive oil
2 cloves garlic, peeled and sliced
1 tbsp crushed baby capers
1½ tsp dried chilli flakes
zest and juice 1 lemon
400 g/14 oz rocket, roughly torn
75 g/3 oz Parmesan cheese, grated
sea salt flakes, freshly ground black pepper

Bring a large pan of water to the boil. Add the pasta and cook following the packet instructions until *al dente*. Heat the oil in a large saucepan, add the garlic and capers and fry for 1 minute. Add the chillies, lemon zest and juice to the pan and cook for another minute. Drain the pasta, then add it to the garlic mixture with the rocket and Parmesan. Toss everything together to combine, season well and serve.

Top tip:

Rocket, which is somewhere between a herb and a salad leaf, has a wonderful peppery flavour. It is in season from May to October.

Marinated salmon

Choose a really fresh salmon and bring it out of the fridge 20 minutes before eating.

Serves: 4
Preparation time: 15 minutes (plus 30 minutes–2 hours marinating time)

450 g/1 lb raw salmon, skinned and thinly sliced
3 tbsp extra virgin olive oil, plus extra for drizzling
1 tbsp vinegar
juice of ½ lemon
2 spring onions, trimmed and finely sliced
handful fresh herbs, such as dill, chervil and parsley

Lay the fish slices on four serving plates. Mix together the oil, vinegar, lemon juice and onions and season. Pour the dressing over the fish and refrigerate for 30 minutes (or longer, if you prefer it slightly more 'cooked'). Remove from the fridge, scatter over the herbs and drizzle a little oil over the top.

Top tip:

Salmon is a fresh water fish in season from May to August. It is a good source of protein, niacin, phosphorous and potassium. Canned salmon is also a good source of calcium because of the soft edible bones it contains.

Creamy smoked mackerel

I defy anyone to tell me they do not like this recipe. It works really well served with the Watercress, orange and fennel salad (see page 93).

Serves: 4
Preparation time: 15 minutes

3 smoked mackerel fillets, skin removed
1 tbsp creamed horseradish
1–2 tsp wholegrain mustard
125 ml/4 fl oz natural yogurt
2 cloves garlic, peeled and roughly chopped
juice of ½ lemon or lime
freshly ground black pepper
fresh crusty bread and wedges of lime, to serve

Put the mackerel, horseradish, mustard, yogurt, garlic and the lemon juice into a food processor, and purée until smooth. Season with freshly ground black pepper.

Top tip:

Mackerel is an oil-rich fish containing omega-3. It is available fresh as well as smoked (look out for mackerel that is undyed). You can also buy smoked mackerel with a coating of ground black pepper

Marinated herrings

If you marinate the herrings the day before, when it comes to lunch, there is very little to do.

Serves: 4
Preparation time: 20 minutes (plus 24 hours marinating time)

100 ml/3½ fl oz white wine vinegar
100 ml/3½ fl oz water
100 ml/3½ fl oz dry sherry
4 allspice berries
1 bay leaf
6 peppercorns
1 red onion, peeled and sliced
1 tsp golden caster sugar
4 herrings, gutted, boned and filleted
6 sprigs fresh dill
50 g/2 oz lamb's lettuce
25 g/1 oz rocket
extra virgin olive oil, to drizzle
sea salt flakes, freshly ground pepper
soured cream and fresh dill, to serve

Put the first eight ingredients into a small saucepan, bring to the boil and simmer for about 2 minutes. Transfer to a bowl and leave to cool. Cut the herrings diagonally into 2 cm/1½ inch pieces and put into a large bowl. Pour the marinade over the top, scatter over the dill, cover and refrigerate for at least 24 hours. Put the lamb's lettuce and rocket in a bowl, drizzle with oil and season to taste. Divide the leaves between four plates, top with the herrings and spoon a little soured cream on top. Finish with some fresh dill.

Oranges and tarragon with cold meats

Serves: 4
Preparation time: 20 minutes

6 juicy oranges
small handful tarragon leaves
handful chervil, roughly chopped
1 tbsp olive oil
pinch sugar
salt
a selection of cold meats, to serve

Cut the top and bottom off the oranges, then cut the skin away from them, making sure that you remove the white pith as you go. Cut the oranges into segments and put into a bowl. Add the tarragon and chervil and mix together. Drizzle with the oil, add the sugar and salt, and chill. Serve with fish or meats.

Top tips:

Segment the oranges over a bowl to save any juice.

Tarragon is warm, spicy and refined, with a light touch of pepper and anise flavours.

Chervil has a delicate, parsley-like flavour with a hint of aniseed. If you are using chervil in cooked dishes, add it towards the end of cooking to retain its subtle character.

Sardines with watercress

Another easy way to eat for energy.

Serves: 4
Preparation time: 15 minutes

3 x 150 g cans sardines in olive oil, drained
2 tbsp olive oil
2 bay leaves
75 g/3 oz bag fresh watercress
1 red onion, peeled and sliced
pinch cumin seeds, toasted
lemon juice, to taste
sea salt flakes, freshly ground black pepper

Put the sardines in a bowl, pour over the olive oil, add the bay leaves and leave to marinate. Arrange the watercress on four serving plates and top with the sardines. Cut the red onion into wafer-thin slices and scatter over the top. Sprinkle with toasted cumin seeds and season with lemon juice, salt and pepper.

Top tip:

Sardines are small herrings. They are one of the best non-dairy sources of calcium.

Tiger prawns with chilli and garlic

Buckwheat noodles are available from most good supermarkets.

Serves: 4
Preparation time: 20 minutes
Cooking time: about 10 minutes

550 g/1 ¼ lb tiger prawns
300 g/10 oz buckwheat noodles
4 spring onions
½ cucumber, halved and seeded
2 tsp olive oil
1 red chilli, seeded and finely chopped
2 cloves garlic, peeled and chopped
2 tsp toasted sesame oil
2 tsp light soy sauce
2 tbsp dry vermouth
squeeze of lime juice
2 limes, cut into chunks, to serve

Cut a thin line down the backs of the prawns and pull out the black veins. Prepare the noodles following the packet instructions. Cut the spring onions and cucumber into thin strips, and put into a bowl with the noodles. Heat the olive oil in a large frying pan, add the chilli and garlic and fry for a minute. Add the prawns and cook until pink all over. Add the sesame oil, soy sauce and vermouth. Leave to simmer for a couple of minutes. Spoon the noodles into four bowls and top with the prawns. Season the pan juices with a squeeze of lime juice and salt and pepper, to taste. Drizzle over the salads and serve with chunks of lime.

Griddled chicken

Marinating chicken before cooking keeps the meat really tender and juicy. Cooking the chicken on a griddle pan requires very little extra oil. If you do not have a griddle pan, invest in one: they are not expensive and are excellent for cooking poultry, meat, fish, fruits and vegetables.

Serves: 4
Preparation time: 15 minutes (plus 30 minutes marinating time)
Cooking time: 10 minutes

juice of 1 lemon
2 cloves garlic, peeled and finely chopped
1 tsp Dijon mustard
2 tbsp balsamic vinegar
sea salt flakes, freshly ground black pepper
4 chicken breasts
1 tbsp olive oil

Put half of the lemon juice in a small bowl with the garlic, mustard, balsamic vinegar and seasoning. Mix together well. Skin the chicken, put into a strong plastic bag and bash until thin. Add to the marinade, cover and refrigerate for 20 minutes. Heat a griddle pan until really hot, add a drizzle of oil and brush to coat. Cook the chicken breasts for a couple of minutes on each side, until charred and cooked through. Serve with the New potato salad (see page 90).

Pan-fried fresh goat's cheese with roast tomatoes and garlic

This lunch is for those days when you are at home and have time to roast a few tomatoes.

Serves: 4
Preparation time: 20 minutes
Cooking time: 30–40 minutes

3 punnets large fresh cherry tomatoes
1 bulb garlic, broken into cloves (unpeeled)
sea salt flakes, freshly ground black pepper
4 x 100 g goat's cheese
plain flour
olive oil
2 tbsp red wine or balsamic vinegar
200 g/7 oz black olives
handful basil leaves

Preheat the oven to 180°C/350°F/gas mark 4. Score a cross into the top of each tomato, put the tomatoes into a bowl, cover with boiling water and leave for 20 seconds. Drain and peel. Put the tomatoes and garlic into an oiled roasting pan, and season. Roast the tomatoes for 30–40 minutes, or until the tomatoes are wrinkled and the garlic is soft and golden. Cut the cheese into thick slices and coat in a little seasoned flour. Heat a little oil in a frying pan and fry the cheese until golden on both sides. Divide the cheese between four warm plates and top with the roasted tomatoes and garlic. Drizzle over the cooking juices and vinegar. Scatter over the olives and basil and serve.

Sweet and spicy glazed chicken

Try always to buy organic chicken.

Serves: 4
Preparation time: 25 minutes (plus at least 15 minutes marinating time)
Cooking time: 10 minutes

4 spring onions, finely sliced
2 tbsp soy sauce
2 tbsp sweet chilli sauce
2.5 cm/1 inch piece fresh root ginger, peeled and grated
1 clove garlic, peeled and crushed
175 g/6 oz redcurrant jelly
5 skinless chicken breasts
fresh coriander, roughly chopped
fresh green salad, to serve

Put the spring onions, soy sauce, sweet chilli sauce, ginger, garlic and redcurrant jelly into a bowl and mix well. Slice the chicken into thin strips, add the strips to the jelly mixture, cover and put into the fridge for at least 15 minutes, preferably longer. Thread the chicken on to skewers and cook under a hot grill for 5 minutes on each side, or until the chicken is cooked in the centre. Scatter over fresh coriander and serve with a green salad.

Chicken with cherries

This is a lunch for the short cherry season. It's a lovely, fresh combination and works really well on its own or with a large green salad. This is also delicious using grapes instead of cherries.

Serves: 4
Preparation time: 20 minutes

4 cooked chicken breasts, skin removed
175 g/6 oz fresh cherries, stoned
6 tbsp soured cream
2 tbsp tarragon vinegar or lemon juice
2 tbsp mayonnaise
2 tbsp roughly chopped fresh tarragon
sea salt flakes, freshly ground black pepper
mixed baby leaf salad, to serve

Slice the chicken breasts thinly and arrange on four plates. Roughly chop the stoned cherries and put into a bowl. In another bowl mix the soured cream, vinegar or lemon juice, mayonnaise, tarragon and season to taste. Stir in the cherries. Top the chicken with the cherry mixture and a few fresh tarragon leaves. Serve with a large mixed baby leaf salad.

Top tip:

Cherries are available for a short time from June to August. To stone cherries split the fruit with the point of a knife then prise out the stones. There are three main types of cherry: sweet, semi-sweet/dessert cherries and sour/morello cherries which are only suitable for cooking.

A few sandwiches

Roasted pepper focaccia

This quantity serves 4 people, and is an ideal sandwich to make when friends drop in for a quick lunch.

Serves: 3–4
Preparation time: 20 minutes
Cooking time: 25 minutes

2 red peppers, halved
2 yellow peppers, halved
1 focaccia loaf or 4 small focaccia loaves
few handfuls fresh rocket leaves
sea salt flakes, freshly ground black pepper

for the dressing:
2 tbsp balsamic vinegar
4 tbsp extra virgin olive oil
1 clove garlic, peeled and finely chopped

Preheat the oven to 180°C/350°F/gas mark 4. Preheat a grill to high, then grill the peppers until black all over. Put into a plastic bag (the steam helps to loosen the skin) and leave to cool for 10 minutes. Remove their skins and seeds. Put all of the dressing ingredients into a screw-top jar and shake well. Cut the focaccia in half, spread a little dressing on to each half and cover the bottom half with the peppers. Top the peppers with as much rocket as you can pack into the sandwich and drizzle with the remaining dressing. Season to taste and cover with the focaccia lid. Transfer to a baking sheet and cover with foil. Bake in the preheated oven for 15 minutes. Serve immediately.

Roasted aubergine, tomatoes and pesto in a baguette

Serves: 3–4
Preparation time: 20 minutes
Cooking time: 15–20 minutes

425 g/15 oz aubergines, thickly sliced
1½ tbsp extra virgin olive oil
2 garlic cloves, peeled
sea salt flakes, freshly ground black pepper
1 tbsp balsamic vinegar
1 French baguette
90 g/3½ oz pesto (from a deli or see page 85)
225 g/8 oz tomatoes, thickly sliced
125 g/4 oz cheese, such as fontina or provolone, thinly sliced
a few lettuce leaves

Preheat the oven to 180°C/350°F/gas mark 4. Put the aubergines into a bowl and toss with the oil, garlic and a few pinches of freshly ground black pepper. Lay the aubergine on a roasting tray and bake for 15–20 minutes, until soft. Remove from the oven and brush the aubergine with balsamic vinegar. Cut the baguette in half, brush both sides with the pesto and lay the aubergine over the top. Follow with an overlapping layer of tomatoes and cheese and season well. Scatter the lettuce over the top and sandwich the baguette together.

Top tip:

Aubergine, otherwise known as eggplant, is available all year round.

Basil aïoli, tomatoes, mozzarella and rocket in granary toast

Serves: 4
Preparation time: 15 minutes

8 slices fresh granary bread
200 g/7 oz mozzarella, thickly sliced
8 ripe tomatoes, thickly sliced
200 g/7 oz fresh rocket leaves

for the basil aïoli:
90 ml/3½ fl oz light and fruity olive oil
50 g/2 oz fresh basil, roughly chopped
1 egg yolk
1½ tsp champagne vinegar
pinch sea salt flakes, freshly ground black pepper
1 garlic clove, peeled and finely chopped

Make the basil aïoli; put the olive oil and basil into a blender and purée. Whisk the egg yolk with a few drops of vinegar until the colour begins to lighten, whisk in the basil oil, drop by drop at first, then a little faster as the mixture thickens and begins to emulsify. Season well and add the remaining vinegar. Spread basil aïoli on to the slices of granary bread, cover four with the sliced mozzarella, followed by the tomatoes and fresh rocket leaves. Top each with the other four slices of bread and cut each sandwich in half.

Avocado with yogurt, lime and red onions

This combination works really well – it's very fresh and the zingy flavours make it a great summer sandwich. If you want to add a little more protein to the sandwich, add a few chunks of tuna or a couple of slices of fresh turkey.

Serves: 4
Preparation time: 10 minutes

3 avocados
juice of ½ lime
65 ml/2 fl oz mayonnaise
65 ml/2 fl oz natural yogurt
sea salt flakes, freshly ground black pepper
8 slices fresh bread – this would be particularly good on focaccia (especially an olive focaccia)
½ red onion, peeled and chopped

Halve the avocados, remove their stones and scoop out the flesh into a bowl. Squeeze in the juice of half a lime, add the mayonnaise and yogurt and beat until smooth, then season to taste. Spread on to four pieces of focaccia, scatter the red onion over the top, season and cover with another slice of bread. Cut in half and serve.

Top tip:

Natural yogurt is a good source of calcium and protein.

Alfalfa sprouts with spicy tomato salsa and houmous

A herb or tomato bread would work really well with this sandwich. Alfalfa sprouts are available from most large supermarkets or health food shops.

Serves: 4
Preparation time: 10 minutes

4 wholemeal rolls or 8 slices bread, such as a herb or tomato bread
150 g/5 oz houmous (see page 123 or buy a pot)
225 g/8 oz alfalfa sprouts or cress
1 tsp chilli sauce
125 g /4 oz tomato salsa (see page 152)

Cut the rolls in half and spread the houmous between the bottom halves. Top with the alfalfa sprouts. Mix the chilli sauce into the salsa and spoon on top. Cover with the lids of the rolls.

Top tips:

Alfalfa sprouts have a rich supply of chlorophyll and amino acids and are said to be one of the most nutritionally valuable plants that we can eat.

For oven-roasted sprouts, put three to four day old wheat, barley or soya bean sprouts on a baking tray and sprinkle with sea salt or vegetable bouillon powder. Bake for 15 minutes in a moderate oven. They become crunchy and are delicious scattered over salads.

Spicy guacamole with roasted vegetables

The pungent ingredients added to this guacomole really enhance the flavour of the avocado and it's a great contrast in texture to the roasted vegetables. You really don't need any butter or mayo in this sandwich – it's perfect as it is. It would be delicious made with a crusty bread such as ciabatta.

Serves: 4
Preparation time: 20 minutes

2 cloves garlic, peeled
2 ripe avocados
1 fresh red chilli, seeded and chopped
juice of half a lemon
2 plum tomatoes, finely chopped
1 spring onion, finely chopped
1 tsp Tabasco
sea salt flakes, freshly ground black pepper
2 tbsp roughly chopped coriander
8 slices bread, such as ciabatta
selection of roasted vegetables (see page 157 or buy from a deli)

Crush the garlic and put into a bowl with the peeled and stoned avocados. Add the chilli, lemon juice, tomato, onion, Tabasco, salt, pepper and coriander. Mash together well, as chunky or as smooth as you like. Spread between all eight slices of the bread. Divide the roasted vegetables between four slices of the avocado-topped bread and top with the remaining slices of bread. Cut in half and serve.

4 Mid-afternoon boosts and pre-dinner nibbles

Mid-afternoon boosts and pre-dinner nibbles

If you are looking for something just that little bit more satisfying, try one of the following snacks. They are quick to make and easy to eat at any time, anywhere.

Avoid eating too many sweet foods in the middle of the afternoon, which can cause your blood sugar and energy level to rise and then quickly fall. Take a look at the following ideas for quick and tasty snacks which will help to keep your energy level constant until supper.

Very quick mid-afternoon boosts

- Toast sunflower and pumpkin seeds and take a bag to work.

Dips/spreads

- Whizz together smoked salmon or poached fresh salmon with curd cheese and lemon juice in a food processor, and serve with toasts.
- Black olive spread is delicious for dipping in fingers of bread or toast.
- Tahini (a paste made from toasted sesame seeds) works well just drizzled over bread or toast. Alternatively spread cashew nut butter on to warm toast.
- Wrap prosciutto around bread sticks and dip into houmus or guacamole (see pages 123 and 124).

Quick ideas with bread

- Toppings for breads – choose whole grains and organic breads and speciality loaves with tomatoes, olives and onions etc. as they are packed with flavour and need less topping to make into a tasty snack. Top with a variety of ingredients, such as aubergine spread, grilled artichokes, peppers, mushrooms or sprouted mung beans with avocado.
- Always try to have a few delicious ingredients, such as fresh crusty bread, a jar of roasted peppers, juicy vine-ripened tomatoes and a pot of basil growing on your windowsill. All you need to do then is to combine these ingredients and you have a delicious quick snack at any time of the day.
- Spring onion sandwich; spread a little olive spread on to two slices bread, top one slice with fresh spring onions, and scatter lots of fresh parsley over the other slice. Cut into small squares and enjoy.
- Cut a piece of ciabatta in half, spread a little olive spread on to the insides and fill with as much watercress as is possible. Squeeze the two pieces together, cut in half, admire the pretty layers of watercress and enjoy.
- Alternate slices of pear with avocado and drizzle with blue cheese dressing.
- Sardines are a source of essential fatty acids and zinc (both needed to feed our brains). Mash into a sandwich with a squeeze of lemon and a few slices of cucumber.
- Spread a thick layer of creamy avocado on to lightly toasted whole wheat bread and drizzle over a mixture of shallot, balsamic vinegar and olive oil. Just before you eat, scatter over lots of roughly chopped fresh coriander.

Sweet snack

- Whizz a bag of frozen berries in a food processor with soya ice cream, or crush and mix with a sorbet and serve in wine glasses for a fruity sensation.

Versatile nibbles

Olives with orange, herbs and garlic

This combination of ingredients is sublime.

Serves: 4
Preparation time: 5 minutes (plus marinating time)

340 g jar juicy black olives
75 ml/3 fl oz extra virgin olive oil
2 garlic cloves, peeled and roughly chopped
3 strips of orange zest
handful fresh herbs, such as tarragon or parsley

Combine the olives, oil, garlic, orange zest and herbs in a bowl. Leave to marinate for a couple of days. Serve with cocktail sticks.

Olives with rosemary and garlic

Make sure you always choose the big juicy Kalamata olives.

Serves: 4
Preparation time: 5 minutes (plus marinating time)

340 g jar Kalamata olives
4 sprigs of fresh rosemary
75 ml/3 fl oz extra virgin olive oil
3 garlic cloves, peeled
sea salt flakes, freshly ground black pepper

Put the olives and garlic in a jar. Stand the rosemary upright among the olives. Half fill the jar with olive oil and leave to marinate for at least three hours.

Hot chilli olives

We rarely eat olives warm, however it makes a pleasant change.

Serves: 4
Preparation time: 5 minutes
Cooking time: 3 minutes

340 g jar large black olives
1 tbsp olive oil
2 red chillies

Bash the olives with a rolling pin, or something hard and flat, to remove the stones. Heat the olive oil in a large wok, add the chillies and fry for a minute. Add the olives, toss together over the heat for a couple of minutes, then serve warm.

Spicy popcorn

It is important to use a heavy-based saucepan (or frying pan) to prevent the popcorn from burning. You also need a tight-fitting lid so that the popcorn remains in the pan until it has popped.

Serves: 2–3
Preparation time: 5 minutes
Cooking time: 10–15 minutes (for a few batches)

1 tbsp vegetable oil
85 g/3 oz corn kernels
2 tbsp olive oil
sea salt flakes, freshly ground black pepper
pinch cayenne pepper and paprika

Heat the vegetable oil until hot in a frying pan. Add the kernels in a single layer. Cover the pan. Listen to the pan and when the kernels begin to pop, turn the heat down and shake gently. When the popping stops, remove the pan from the heat, and tip the corn into a dish. Add the olive oil, seasoning, cayenne pepper and paprika, to taste, then serve.

Top tip:

If you prefer a sweet version, add cinnamon, instead of cayenne and paprika, and a sprinkling of sugar instead of salt.

Chilli peanuts

There are many variations that can be made on this theme. Have fun experimenting with different spices.

Preparation time: 5 minutes
Cooking time: 12 minutes

150 g/5 oz raw peanuts, shelled
½ tsp peanut oil
¼ tsp paprika
¼ tsp cayenne pepper
¼ tsp sea salt flakes

Preheat the oven to 170°C/325°F/gas mark 3. In a small bowl, toss the nuts with the oil, spices and salt. Roast them on a baking sheet for about 12 minutes, until they smell nutty. Cool and store in an airtight container.

Top tip:

Peanuts are legumes, not nuts at all. They are a good source of protein, niacin, phosphorous, potassium and, although they are cholesterol free, they do contain fat.

Soy nuts

Serves: 2–3
Preparation time: 5 minutes
Cooking time: 5 minutes

1 tbsp vegetable oil
1–2 tsp Kashmiri chilli powder (Bart Spices)
100 g/3½ oz brazil nuts
100 g/3½ oz almonds
3–4 tbsp soy sauce (or to your personal taste)
sea salt flakes (optional)

Heat the oil in a wok or large frying pan, add the chilli powder and cook for a minute. Add the nuts and toss to coat with the oil and chilli and fry for a minute. Add the soy to the pan; it will sizzle as it hits the hot nuts. Sauté over a high heat for 3 minutes or until the pan is dry, stirring frequently so that the nuts do not burn. Toss a few sea salt flakes over and leave to cool on kitchen paper (to drain any excess oil). Serve.

Top tip:

If you find that the nuts are not spicy enough, heat a little more oil, add more chilli powder and return the nuts to the pan. Cook for a few minutes, tossing the nuts to prevent them from burning.

Toasted seeds

Experiment with the quantity of cayenne pepper until you get them to the correct heat.

Serves: 2–3
Preparation time: 5 minutes
Cooking time: 15–25 minutes

125 g/4 oz sunflower seeds
125 g/4 oz pumpkin seeds
sea salt flakes
1 tsp cayenne pepper
2 tbsp light and fruity olive oil

Preheat the oven to 190°C/ 375°F/ gas mark 5.
Put the seeds in a roasting dish, sprinkle over sea salt flakes and cayenne pepper and toss everything together. Drizzle over a little olive oil and roast in the preheated oven for 15–25 minutes, turning occasionally to ensure the seeds brown evenly; they are ready when the seeds are golden. Alternatively, toss the seeds in the sea salt and cayenne pepper and dry fry them in a frying pan over a gentle heat until golden.

Dips/spreads for vegetable sticks, breads or salads

Fresh herb and lemon juice

This makes a refreshing change to creamy dips for vegetables and crisps. In fact it is also a delicious sauce for hot vegetables, especially drizzled over mashed potato or steamed asparagus spears.

Serves: 2–3
Preparation time: 5 minutes
Cooking time: 10 minutes

100 ml/3½ fl oz extra virgin olive oil
25 g/1 oz unsalted butter
2 cloves garlic, peeled and finely chopped
1 small bunch parsley, roughly chopped
1 small bunch of coriander, roughly chopped
selection of fresh vegetables, such as baby beets, radicchio, fennel, carrots, red and yellow peppers (choose a selection of seasonal vegetables of different shapes and colours)

Heat the oil and butter over a low heat until the butter melts. Add the garlic and cook, stirring frequently until tender, for about 10 minutes, without allowing the oil to bubble. Add the herbs and serve immediately with a selection of wonderful vegetables.

Top tip:

Vary your choice of bread if you are going to serve these dips with breads, such as organic whole grain bagels, pitta, rye crisp or chapatis. Alternatively, serve with organic tortilla chips.

Houmous

Another simple dish that combines a few fresh flavours to make a tasty and light dip without turning the oven on. Versions of this recipe often use a large amount of oil, but to keep this light and hip-friendly, I've used a combination of oil, lemon juice and water.

Serves: 4–6 (depending on how hungry your guests are)
Preparation time: 10 minutes

2 x 420 g cans chickpeas, drained and rinsed
2 garlic cloves, peeled and chopped
juice of 1 lemon
3 tbsp olive oil
50 ml/2 fl oz water
sea salt flakes, freshly ground black pepper
handful fresh mint, roughly chopped
raw vegetables or pitta bread, to serve

Put the chickpeas, garlic and lemon juice in a blender and process until smooth. Gradually add the oil and water in a thin stream, keeping the motor running. Purée until the chickpeas are smooth, and season with salt and freshly ground black pepper. Transfer to a serving bowl, scatter the mint over the top and serve with a selection of raw vegetables or pitta bread.

Fresh green salad with Parmesan crisps

Creamy fish curry with cucumber salsa

Brown sugar and hazelnut meringues

Creamy lemon parfait

Guacamole

A dip based on a dish from Mexico. Perfect for serving with raw vegetables or Spicy chips (see page 128).

Serves: 4
Preparation time: 15 minutes

2 cloves garlic, peeled
2 ripe avocados (Hass)
1 fresh red chilli, seeded and chopped
juice of ½ lemon
2 plum tomatoes, finely chopped
1 spring onion, finely chopped
1 tsp Tabasco
sea salt flakes, freshly ground black pepper
2 tbsp roughly chopped coriander

Crush the garlic and put into a bowl. Cut the avocados in half, remove the stones and scoop the flesh into a bowl with the garlic. Add the chilli, lemon juice, tomato, onion, Tabasco, salt, pepper and coriander. Mash together well – as chunky or as smooth as you like.

Avocado with limes

This is a variation of the Guacamole recipe.

Serves: 2–3
Preparation time: 10 minutes

4 avocados (Hass)
juice of 2 limes
3 spring onions, finely chopped
1 bunch fresh coriander, roughly chopped
1 red chilli, seeded and finely chopped
sea salt flakes, freshly ground black pepper

Cut the avocados in half, remove the stones and scoop the flesh into a bowl. Add half of the lime juice, spring onions, coriander and chilli. Season to taste; you may need to add extra lime juice.

Top tip:

Avocados may have a high fat content, but they also contain substantial amounts of potassium and vitamins. They are low in sodium and contain zero cholesterol.

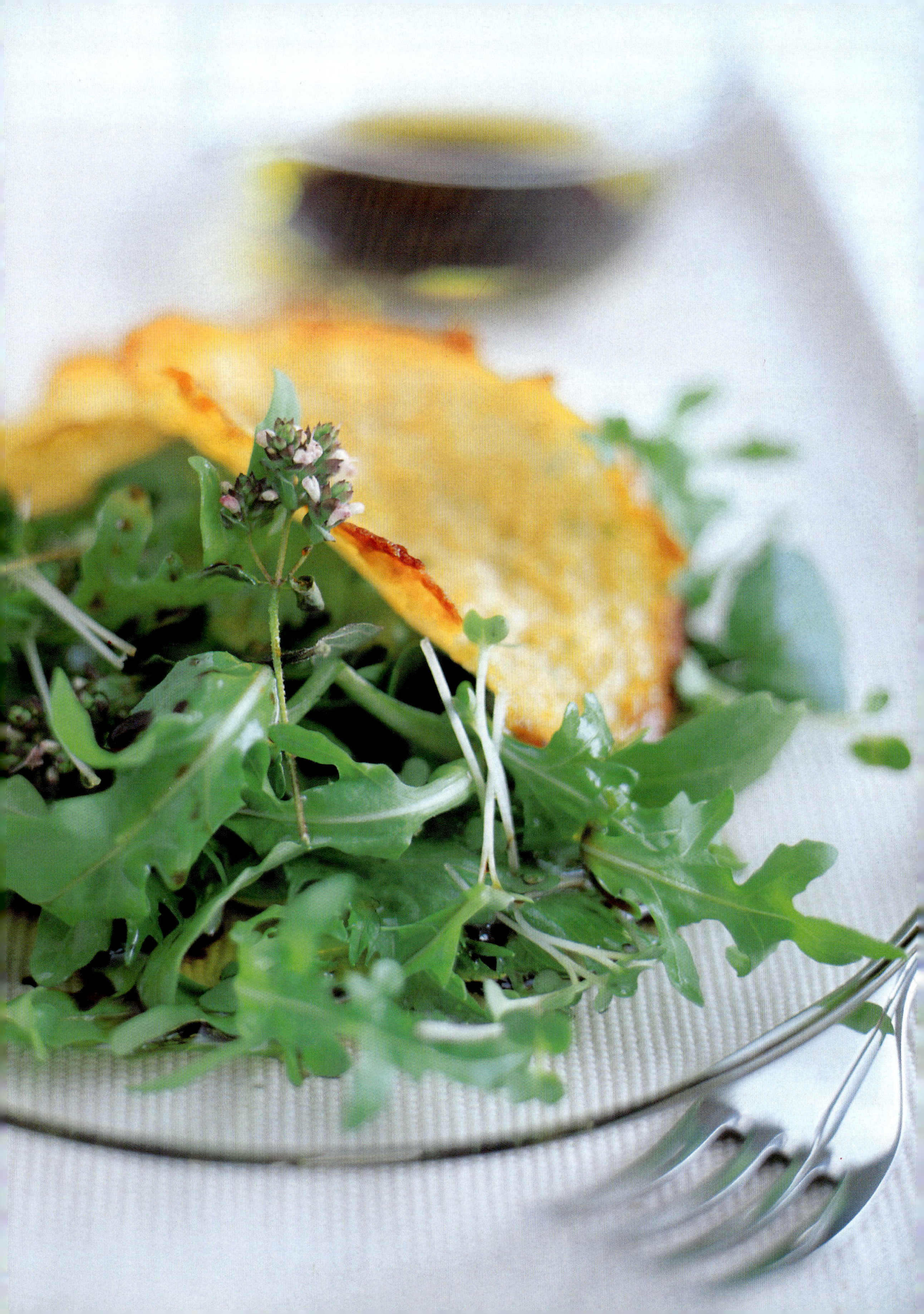

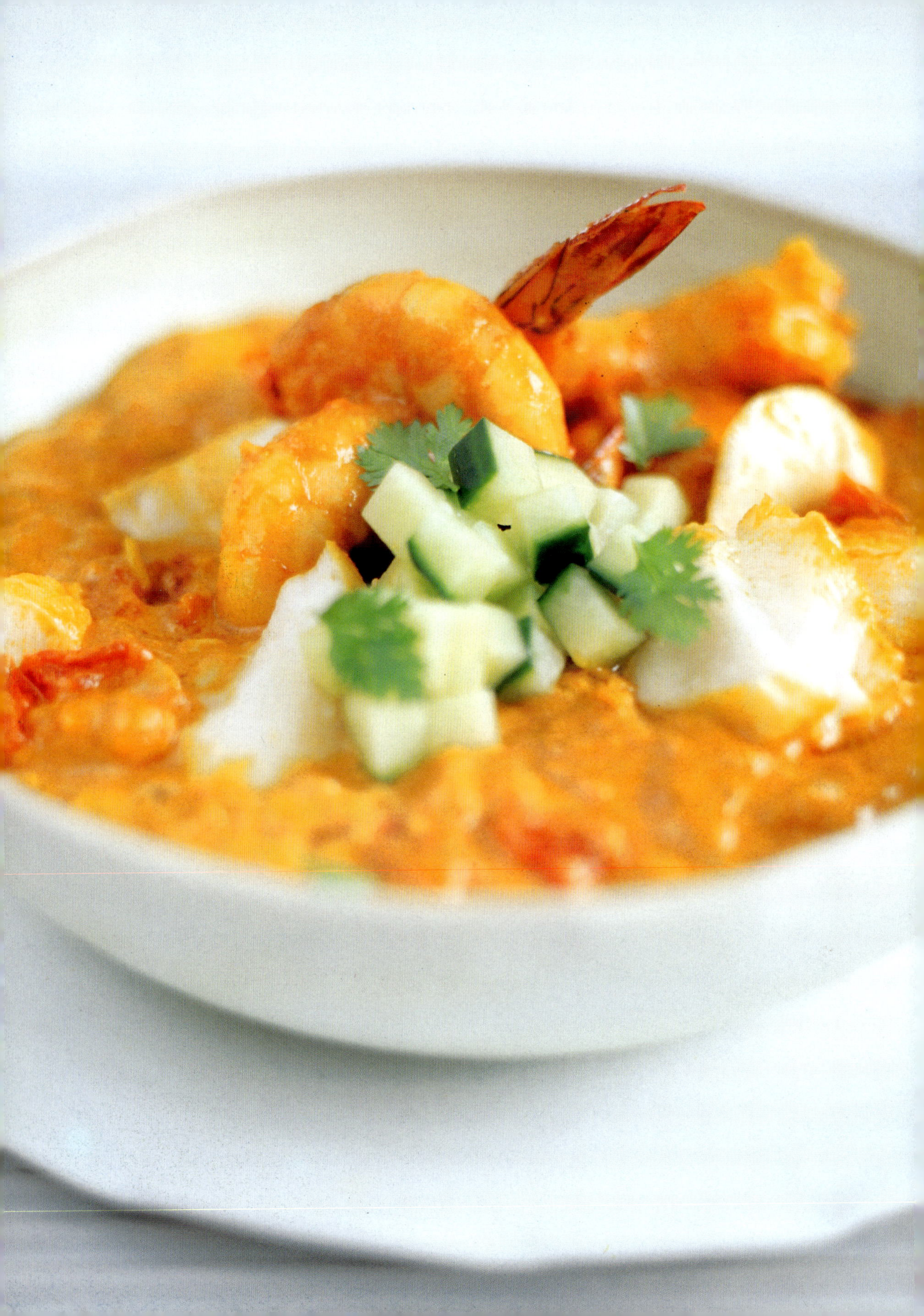

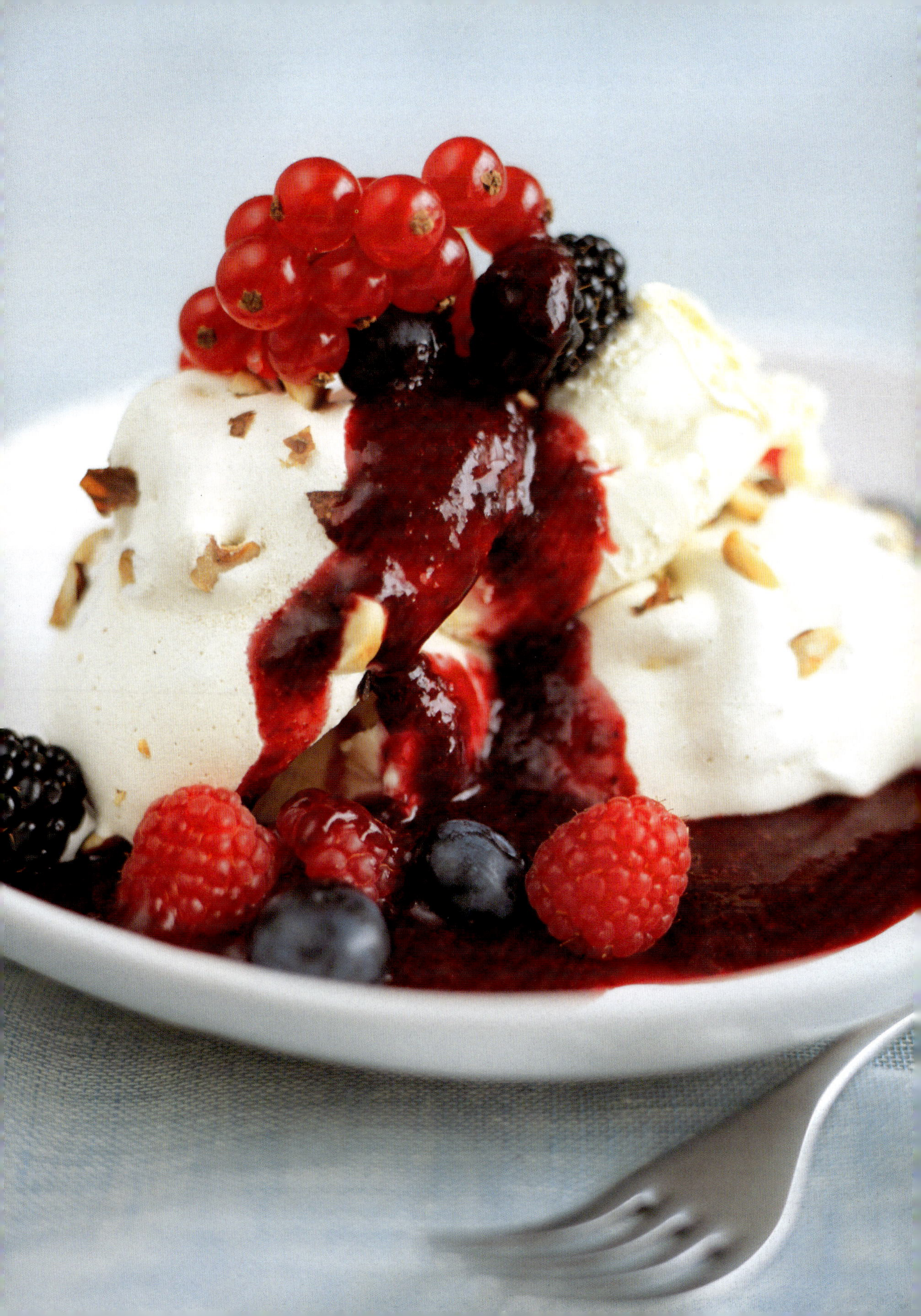

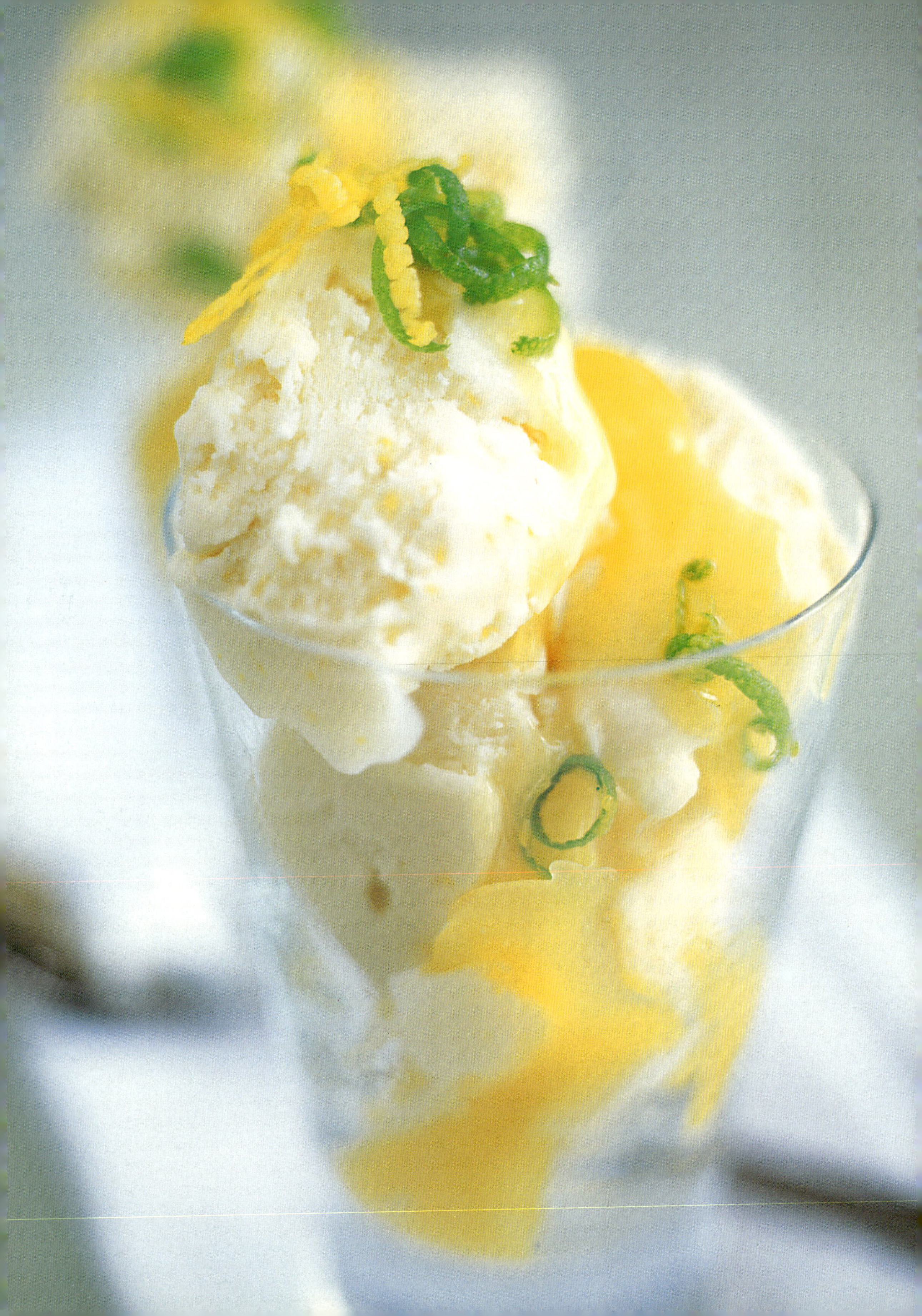

Roasted aubergine and bean dip

I have made this to serve 4, rather than 2–3, as you do need to turn the oven on and make a little effort.

Serves: 4
Preparation time: 15–20 minutes
Cooking time: 50 minutes

2 aubergines, halved
2 cloves garlic
185 g/6½ oz cannellini beans
75 ml/3 fl oz olive oil
juice of 1 lemon
pinch cumin seeds, toasted and ground
sea salt flakes, freshly ground black pepper
handful fresh parsley, roughly chopped
1 packet fresh mint, roughly chopped
raw vegetables or warm bread, to serve

Preheat the oven to 200°C/400°F/gas mark 6. Put the aubergines and garlic into a roasting dish, drizzle with 25 ml/1 fl oz oil, and roast for 50 minutes until the skins are well charred and the flesh is soft. Peel the skins from the aubergine and garlic, put the flesh into a food processor and whizz until smooth. Add the beans, oil, lemon juice and cumin and whizz again until smooth. Season to taste and stir in the herbs. Serve with warmed bread or raw vegetables.

Beetroot and yogurt

I was first served this dip at a barbeque party. It was served with succulent barbecued chicken, more as an accompaniment than a dip, and was absolutely delicious.

Serves: 4–6
Preparation time: 20 minutes

¼ cucumber
200 g/7 oz cooked beetroot
1 tbsp extra virgin olive oil
1 tsp white wine vinegar
150 g/5 oz organic yogurt
sea salt flakes, freshly ground black pepper
½ shallot, peeled and finely chopped
handful each fresh dill and mint, roughly chopped

Cut the cucumber in half, lengthways, and scoop out the seeds. Slice the flesh into little strips and finely dice. Finely dice the beetroot. Put the oil, vinegar and yogurt into a bowl and whisk together, then season to taste. Add the cucumber and beetroot and mix together; you may like to mash the mixture at this stage to make it slightly less chunky. Add half of the herbs and leave covered in the fridge until required. Serve garnished with the remaining herbs.

Cheese and mint

Dips cannot get simpler than this. If you prefer, try the same dip with a different herb.

Serves: 2–3
Preparation time: 5 minutes

175 g/6 oz medium mature goat's cheese
2 tbsp extra olive oil
freshly ground black pepper
handful fresh mint, roughly chopped

Remove the rind from the cheese and then crumble the cheese into a bowl. Drizzle over the oil, season to taste with black pepper and mash to a coarse paste. Scatter over the fresh mint and serve.

Butter bean paté

This butter bean paté will go with any vegetables; try it with peppers, ripe juicy tomatoes, grated carrot, roasted vegetables or beansprouts.

Serves: 4
Preparation time: 5 minutes

400 g can butter beans
3 tbsp extra virgin olive oil
2 cloves garlic, peeled and crushed
juice of 1 lemon
3 tbsp fresh coriander, roughly chopped
pinch paprika
sea salt flakes, freshly ground black pepper

Put all the paté ingredients in a food processor and whizz until just smooth. The paté will keep in the fridge for 3–4 days.

Spicy peanut sauce with vegetables and toasts

Make this sauce and keep it in the fridge for those snack attack feelings. If you have time, grill a few fresh vegetables to serve with it, or chop up some fresh vegetables and use as a dip. Scatter over extra peanuts and fresh coriander before serving.

Serves: 3–4
Preparation time: 10–15 minutes

1 tbsp coarsely chopped onion
1 large garlic clove, peeled and finely chopped
1 or 2 red jalapeno chillies, seeded
1 tbsp peanut oil
2½ tbsp soy sauce
1 tbsp plus 1 tsp lime juice
2 tbsp light soft brown sugar
1 tsp molasses
125 g/4 oz creamy peanut butter
50 ml/2 fl oz water
¼ tsp cayenne pepper

Put the onion, garlic, chillies, oil, soy and lime juice in a blender or food processor. Blend until smooth, then transfer to a bowl. Whisk in the remaining ingredients.

Quick hot snacks

Hot bacon bites

These are a great snack to have at home and they also make a delicious nibble to serve to friends with drinks before supper.

Serves: 3–4
Preparation time: 10 minutes
Cooking time: 1 hour

20 prunes, dates and figs (in any combination you choose)
10 rashers streaky bacon
Worcestershire sauce, for dipping

Preheat the oven to 200°C/400°F/gas mark 6. Wrap the bacon around the fruit and secure each with a cocktail stick. Bake for 1 hour until the bacon is crisp and the fruit are sticky. Serve with a little bowl of Worcestershire sauce, for dipping.

Top tip:

Prunes are not just dried plums, but a sugary European variety that can be dried, pit and all, without fermenting. They are firmer than other plums, more acidic, but honey-sweet, too. Prunes are quick sources of energy and contain hefty shots of iron, potassium and fibre.

Tapenade toasts

Crisp toasts with a really olive kick.

Serves: 3–4
Preparation time: 20 minutes

2 tbsp capers, rinsed
2 cloves garlic, peeled and roughly chopped
4 anchovy fillets, rinsed
225 g/8 oz black olives, stoned
2 tsp olive oil

for the toasts:
30 ml/1½ fl oz extra virgin olive oil
1 garlic, peeled and finely chopped
12 thin slices baguette
handful fresh parsley, roughly chopped

Preheat the oven to 190°C/375°F/gas mark 5. Pound together the capers, garlic and anchovy fillets in a mortar and pestle and pound until crushed. Add the olives a few at a time, crushing thoroughly, but stop before the mixture becomes slush. Stir in the oil.

To make the toasts, put the oil and garlic into a bowl and mix together. Brush the bread with the oil and arrange on a baking sheet. Toast until crisp and lightly golden, for about 8 minutes. Spread ½ tablespoon of tapenade on to each of the toasts or place a small dollop on to each piece before you eat, and sprinkle with parsley.

Spicy chips

A bowl of chips should be a treat rather than the norm, but when you do make them you need to make sure that they are cooked properly. I fry them for a few minutes, drain and fry quickly again, this way the chips are crisp on the outside and fluffy in the middle.

Serves: 4
Preparation time: 15 minutes
Cooking time: about 15 minutes

900 g/2 lb potatoes
8 tsp cayenne pepper
vegetable oil, for frying
sea salt flakes

Peel and cut the potatoes into thin wedges, then sprinkle with 3 teaspoons of cayenne pepper. Fill a frying pan to a third with vegetable oil and bring up to a good heat. Add a cube of bread and when it browns quickly, it is hot enough. Add half of the potato and fry for 4–5 minutes. Remove and allow the oil to get hot again. Return the chips to the pan for 1 minute, transfer to a plate lined with kitchen paper, then sprinkle with another teaspoon of cayenne and sea salt to taste. Repeat with the remaining potatoes.

Griddled sweet potato

Serves: 4
Preparation time: 15 minutes
Cooking time: 30 minutes

4 sweet potatoes
olive oil, for brushing
sea salt flakes, freshly ground black pepper
tomato relish, to serve

Gently scrub the potatoes to clean. Bring a large pan of water to the boil and cook the potatoes for about 20 minutes until tender; test with a sharp knife, it should just go through the middle. Drain and leave to cool. Cut the potato into thick slices, brush with a little oil, then sprinkle with sea salt flakes and freshly ground black pepper. Heat a griddle pan until hot and griddle the potato slices for a couple of minutes on each side. Serve with a Chunky tomato sauce (see page 106).

Top tip:

The best sweet potato that we can get is orange-fleshed and usually comes from South Africa or Israel.

Warm tomato scones

Enjoy hot scones straight from the oven dipped in olive oil and served with a chunk of Parmesan cheese.

Serves: 4
Preparation time: 15 minutes
Cooking time: 15 minutes

200 g/7 oz self-raising wholemeal flour
½ tsp baking powder
½ tsp sea salt
50 g/2 oz sun-dried tomatoes, roughly chopped
25 g/1 oz fresh parsley, roughly chopped
4 tbsp extra virgin olive oil
1 medium egg
75 ml/3 fl oz milk
25 g/1 oz Parmesan cheese, grated
extra virgin olive oil and Parmesan cheese, to serve

Sift the flour, baking powder and salt into a bowl; add the grains from the sieve. Stir in the sun-dried tomato and herbs, then make a well in the middle. Mix together the oil, egg and milk and pour into the well. Mix everything together, but do not beat. Drop 10 small spoonfuls on to a baking sheet, sprinkle with the grated cheese and bake for 12–14 minutes until golden brown and cooked through. Eat warm with olive oil for dipping and a chunk of Parmesan cheese.

Mushrooms with herbs

Serves: 2
Preparation time: 10 minutes
Cooking time: 5–8 minutes

4 large field mushrooms
handful fresh parsley and mint, roughly chopped
2 cloves garlic, peeled and finely chopped
2 tbsp extra virgin olive oil
sea salt flakes, freshly ground black pepper

Wipe the mushrooms clean and place them, gill side up, in a baking tray. Mix the herbs, garlic and oil in a bowl and season well. Drizzle the herb mixture over the mushrooms and grill for 5–8 minutes, basting with the juices as they cook.

Top tip:

Wipe or brush mushrooms to clean them rather than washing them with water as they act like a sponge and absorb the moisture.

Tiny pasta with fresh herbs

If you or the family get really hungry, cook some quick pasta and make this even quicker sauce.

Serves: 2
Preparation time: 10 minutes
Cooking time: 10 minutes

150 g/5 oz pasta
150 ml/5 fl oz thick Greek yogurt
handful fresh herbs, such as tarragon, parsley or dill, roughly chopped
1 tbsp lemon juice
sea salt flakes, freshly ground black pepper

Bring a large pan of water to the boil and cook the pasta according to the packet instructions then drain. Put the yogurt into a saucepan, add all of the fresh herbs and mix in the lemon juice. Season well, add the pasta, mix together and serve.

Things to go on bread/toast

Salmon with lime and yogurt

This is delicious on bread as an open sandwich or served as a salad. Make sure you use really fresh salmon.

Serves: 2
Preparation time: 10 minutes

125 g/4 oz raw salmon (it must be very fresh)
juice of 1 lime
2 tbsp yogurt
sea salt flakes, freshly ground black pepper
bunch watercress
¼ cucumber, very thinly sliced

Chop up the salmon into small pieces, put into a bowl, add the lime juice, yogurt and season well. Divide the watercress between pieces of bread or toast, followed by the cucumber. Top with the salmon mixture.

Top tip:

Salmon is a fairly fatty fish, but most of the fat is unsaturated. Fresh salmon is a good source of niacin, phosphorous and potassium.

Open avocado and tomato sandwiches

Botanically avocado is a fruit, like the tomato, however it is often eaten like a vegetable. In Brazil, they are mashed with sugar and eaten as a dessert. If you ever want to speed up the ripening process of avocado, put the fruit into a brown paper bag.

Serves: 2
Preparation time: 10 minutes
Cooking time: 2 minutes

2 slices granary bread
1 avocado (Hass)
4 ripe tomatoes, sliced
2 shallots, peeled and finely chopped
2 tbsp balsamic vinegar
4 tbsp extra virgin olive oil
handful fresh coriander, roughly chopped

Toast the bread. Cut the avocado in half, remove the stone and peel the fruit. Slice the avocado and tomatoes and arrange on top of the toast. Mix together the dressing ingredients and drizzle over the avocado. Scatter over the coriander and enjoy.

Sweet nibbles

Tomatoes with chives

This is so easy and such a healthy, delicious snack to nibble in the middle of the afternoon.

Serves: 2
Preparation time: 10 minutes

4–6 medium/large ripe tomatoes
1 shallot, peeled and finely chopped
1 small bunch chives
4 tbsp olive oil
2 tsp lemon juice
sea salt flakes, freshly ground black pepper
fresh bread, to serve

Cut the tomatoes in thin slices and lay them over a platter or large plate. Finely chop the shallot and scatter over the tomatoes. Snip the chives over the top, mix together the oil and lemon juice, season well and drizzle over the tomatoes. Leave at room temperature for a few minutes until ready to serve with fresh bread to mop up the juices.

Fast berry ice cream

This has got to be the quickest ice cream yet. All right, it is not technically an ice cream, but it certainly tastes and looks like one. It is an ideal treat to give to children: simply serve it in cones and they will never know the difference (just remember to omit the liqueur!).

Serves: 4
Preparation time: 10 minutes

450 g/1 lb frozen berries
125 g/4 oz thick Greek yogurt
125 g/4 oz crème fraiche
25 g/1 oz golden icing sugar
2 tbsp berry liqueur of your choice, such as Crème de Cassis (optional), plus extra for serving
4 sprigs fresh mint, to serve

Take the berries out of the freezer 10 minutes before you are ready to make the dessert. Reserve a handful of berries, put the rest into a food processor, add the yogurt, crème fraiche, icing sugar and liqueur, if using, and purée until smooth. Spoon into glasses or bowls, drizzle each with a little berry liqueur, scatter over a few reserved berries and finish with sprigs of fresh mint.

Banana, fig and honey cake

Preparation time: 10 minutes
Cooking time: 30 minutes

3 eggs (medium)
175 g/6 oz soft brown sugar
200 ml/7 fl oz sunflower oil
175 ml/6 fl oz milk
125 g/4 oz plain flour
125 g/4 oz wholemeal flour
½ tsp bicarbonate soda
1 tsp cinnamon
large pinch nutmeg
1 tsp mixed spice
2 bananas, mashed
250 g/9 oz figs or dates, stoned and chopped
3 tbsp honey, to serve – for the top

Preheat the oven to 190°C/375°F/gas mark 5. Butter and flour an 8-inch cake tin. Put everything into a bowl, except the bananas and figs or dates, and whisk until mixed together. Stir in the mashed bananas and chopped figs or dates. Spoon into the tin and bake for 45 minutes–1 hour or until a skewer comes out clean. Make holes over the cake with a fork and pour over honey to serve.

Chocolate and berry cake

This is for those times when you really need something sweet and preferably tasting of chocolate. Serve a slice with a few fresh berries and a large dollop of thick and creamy Greek yogurt.

Serves: 6
Preparation time: 15 minutes
Cooking time: 40 minutes

250g/9 oz self-raising flour
85g/3oz cocoa powder
3 tsp baking powder
250g/9oz golden caster sugar
1½ tsp vanilla extract (optional)
120ml/4 fl oz corn oil
360ml/12 fl oz organic milk
125 g/4½ oz frozen mixed berries
55 g/2oz Brazil and pecan nuts, toasted and chopped
1 tsp golden icing sugar, to serve

Preheat the oven to 180°C/350F/gas mark 4. Grease an 8-inch cake tin and line the base with greaseproof paper. Sift the flour, cocoa and baking powder into a bowl and add the sugar, vanilla if used, oil and milk. Mix with an electric whisk to a thick batter-like consistency. Add the frozen mixed berries and toasted nuts. Pour into the tin. Cook for 45–55 minutes until cooked on the outside and still slightly squidgy in the middle. Turn out on to a wire rack to cool. Alternatively, serve warm. Dust with golden icing sugar before serving.

5

Suppers

Suppers

Eat a good few hours before you go to bed so that when you are asleep your energy is devoted to repairing and rebuilding the cells in your body. If you eat straight before going to sleep, your energy will be directed towards the intestines and digesting the food, and as a result you are less likely to feel refreshed in the morning. Similarly, if you exercise in the evenings, eat a small snack first and supper afterwards; otherwise the energy gained from your supper will not be used to aid digestion.

The recipes in this section are all quite light, and do not require hours of digesting. However, whenever possible, eat at least three hours before sleep. This will help you wake up feeling refreshed and ready to start the new day.

I have kept the starters fresh and tasty to tempt the taste buds rather than overload them with flavours. For example, roasted peppers marinated in their own juices with balsamic vinegar, olive oil and basil are simply delicious served with small pieces of toast and perhaps a wedge of crumbly goat's cheese. Similarly, soft eggs with fresh tomatoes and watercress make a wonderful combination. I also love the simplicity of dishes like grilled asparagus served with a fresh, minty vinaigrette or thin slices of pancetta or prosciutto and shavings of Parmesan.

Take a look at the Mid-afternoon boost chapter to choose a few quick 'nibbles' to serve with drinks. Bowls of green and black olives are very quick and easy to prepare, just add a few herbs and oils for a new flavour sensation. Similarly, a bowl of fresh radishes with a little jug of fresh vinaigrette is just divine with a long, cool refreshing drink. Drizzle the vinaigrette over the radishes and nibble with bread.

Have fun creating these recipes and enjoy them.

Antipasto of peppers

There is nothing quite as delightful as serving a platter of lots of little antipasto for a starter. It looks so pretty and the flavours and textures are just fabulous. You can make a simple dish like this one and then add grilled artichokes, olives, dips, fresh vegetables and breads to make a more substantial starter or lunch.

Serves: 4
Preparation time: 20 minutes
Cooking time: 15 minutes

6 peppers (2 red, 2 yellow, 2 orange)
3 tbsp extra virgin olive oil
juice of 1 lemon
1 clove garlic, peeled and finely chopped
black olives
sea salt flakes, freshly ground black pepper

Cut the peppers in half and put on a baking tray, cut side down. Grill until black all over, turning the peppers around occasionally, for about 15 minutes. Transfer to a plastic bag (the steam helps to loosen the skin) and leave to cool. When cool enough to handle, remove the skins. Slice the peppers into strips. Put the oil, lemon juice, garlic and olives into a bowl, season and mix everything together. Add the peppers and leave to marinate for 30 minutes. Serve at room temperature with fresh bread.

Starters or little nibbles

Barbecued corn with chilli oil

This is a must when you have hot weather. All you need to accompany the corn is some fresh fish and a large bowl of salad to have a complete meal outside.

Serves: 4
Preparation time: 5 minutes
Cooking time: 8–10 minutes

4 corn on the cobs (with husks)
3 tbsp olive oil
1 red chilli, seeded and finely chopped
handful fresh coriander, roughly chopped
sea salt flakes, freshly ground black pepper

Peel the husks back from the corn. Tear out the corn silk and throw away, then pull the husks back over the corn. Moisten the husks with water (this helps to prevent them from burning). Barbeque for 7–8 minutes, turning every few minutes. Mix the oil, chilli and coriander and season. Pull back the husks, drizzle the chilli oil over the corn and eat.

Mushrooms with tapenade

My alternative to garlic mushrooms.

Serves: 4
Preparation time: 15 minutes
Cooking time: 10–15 minutes

4 large field mushrooms
4 tsp tapenade
1 clove garlic, peeled and finely chopped
50 g/2 oz goat's cheese
sea salt flakes, freshly ground black pepper
50 g/2 oz fresh Parmesan
handful fresh parsley, roughly chopped

Preheat the oven to 200°C/400°F/gas mark 6. Wipe the mushrooms with a damp cloth, trim off the stalks and place upside down in a baking tray. Put the tapenade, garlic and goat's cheese into a bowl and mix together. Spread the tapenade mixture on to the mushrooms. Sprinkle over the Parmesan and bake in the top of the oven for 10–15 minutes (the mushrooms should be tender and golden on top). Scatter over the parsley and serve.

Top tip:

Field mushrooms should be kept dry when stored as they have a sponge-like density, which absorbs or sweats out moisture. Wrap in a paper towel then store in a paper bag in the salad section of the fridge.

Soft eggs with tomatoes and watercress

Serves: 4
Preparation time: 20 minutes
Cooking time: 15 minutes

450 g/1 lb new potatoes
big bunch fresh watercress, washed and picked through
4 free-range eggs
300 g/11 oz ripe tomatoes (a selection of your choice – I love the Pomodorino tomatoes)
handful of each fresh chervil and parsley, roughly chopped

for the vinaigrette:
4 tbsp extra virgin olive oil
2 tbsp white wine vinegar
1 tbsp Dijon mustard
sea salt flakes, freshly ground black pepper
1 tsp sugar

Bring a pan of water to the boil, add the potatoes and cook until tender (a knife should easily pierce through the flesh), then drain. Put the watercress into a large bowl. Put all of the vinaigrette ingredients into a jar and shake well. Heat a large pan of water and lower the heat just before it starts to simmer. Carefully break the eggs into the water, cover, cook for 1 minute (exactly) and remove from the heat. Leave to stand for 8 minutes. Chop the tomatoes into thin wedges or slices (depending on their size) and add to the watercress with the warm potatoes. Pour over the vinaigrette and toss everything together. Divide between four serving plates. Use a slotted spoon to lift an egg on to each salad. Season well, scatter over some fresh herbs and serve.

Baby asparagus

The Egyptians, Greeks, Romans and Arabs all delighted in asparagus, both as a food and an aphrodisiac. Here, asparagus is served with fresh leaves and a very light vinaigrette, a delightful feast indeed. Incredibly simple, yet always received with praise and thanks, it is a wonderful way to start supper, especially during May and June when asparagus is in season.

Serves: 4
Preparation time: 10 minutes
Cooking time: about 5 minutes

350 g/12 oz asparagus spears
3 sprigs fresh mint
grated zest and juice of 1 lime
3 tbsp extra virgin olive oil
sea salt flakes, freshly ground black pepper
4 handfuls fresh leaves, such as rocket, radicchio, chicory and frisée
handful of each mint and chives, roughly chopped

Bring a pan of water to the boil, add the asparagus and mint, and cook for 3–4 minutes, or until just tender, then drain. Put the lime zest and juice, oil and seasoning into a jar and shake well. Divide the salad leaves between four plates, top with the asparagus and drizzle over the dressing. Scatter over the herbs and serve.

Sesame mushrooms

Serves: 4
Preparation time: 15 minutes
Cooking time: 10 minutes

450 g/1 lb chestnut mushrooms
2 tbsp sesame oil
2 cloves garlic, peeled and crushed
1 tsp Sichuan peppercorns, crushed
freshly ground black pepper
2 tbsp dry sherry
3 tbsp light soy sauce

Wipe the mushrooms and cut into wedges. Heat the oil in a frying pan, add the mushrooms and sauté over a medium heat for 2–3 minutes. Add the garlic and Sichuan peppercorns and cook for a further 2 minutes. Season the mushrooms with pepper, sherry and soy, bring to the boil and cook for 1 minute. Tip into four little bowls and serve with toast.

Top tip:

Dark soy sauce is aged for longer than light soy and it is mixed with molasses. This gives the sauce its stronger flavour and deeper colour. Dark soy is generally added to flavour and colour heartier dishes, whereas light is used for seafood, vegetables, soups and dipping sauces. Japanese soy (Kikkoman, introduced by China), as opposed to Chinese soy, contains more wheat and is fermented for longer than the traditional six months, and this makes it sweeter and less salty.

Fresh leaves with tomatoes and goat's cheese

Make the most of salad leaves and wonderful ingredients such as juicy tomatoes and fresh goat's cheese when they are at their best.

Serves: 4
Preparation time: 15 minutes

for the dressing:
2 tbsp balsamic vinegar
50 ml/2 fl oz extra virgin olive oil
1 garlic clove, peeled and finely chopped
sea salt flakes, freshly ground black pepper
splash sherry vinegar

2 large bunches lettuce leaves, washed
50 g/2 oz watercress, washed
1 tbsp pine nuts, toasted
3 sun-dried tomatoes, finely sliced
50 g/2 oz mild goat's cheese

Put all of the dressing ingredients into a jar and shake well. Tear the leaves and put into a bowl. Add the watercress, pine nuts and tomatoes. Drizzle over the vinaigrette and toss everything together. Crumble in the goat's cheese and season well.

Fresh green salad with Parmesan crisps

Serves: 4
Preparation time: 15 minutes
Cooking time: 5 minutes

for the Parmesan crisps:
75 g/3 oz Parmesan cheese, finely grated
large bunch each of rocket, watercress, baby spinach and mustard cress
1 tbsp fresh herbs, such as chives and marjoram, finely chopped

for the dressing:
4 tbsp extra virgin olive oil
2 tbsp balsamic vinegar
2 tbsp fresh herbs, such as marjoram, roughly chopped
freshly ground black pepper

Heat a grill. Place a sheet of bakewell paper on a baking tray and spoon the Parmesan into small, flat rounds (about 6 cm/2½ inches in diameter). Grill for about 4–5 minutes (the cheese will melt and bubble) until golden. Using a palette knife, transfer the crisps to a cooling rack, bend the edges into the middle to create a pretty curled leaf shape and leave until crisp. Put all of the green leaves and herbs into a large bowl. Put all of the dressing ingredients into a jar and shake well. Pour the dressing over the leaves and toss everything together. Divide between four plates. Top each salad with a few Parmesan crisps, season and serve.

Rocket and beef salad with a horseradish dressing

The fresh green peppery rocket is delicious with thin strips of beef and a sharp horseradish dressing. If you are vegetarian, this salad also works well without the beef.

Serves: 4
Preparation time: 10 minutes

1 red onion, peeled
2 large bunches fresh rocket
handful fresh basil leaves, roughly torn
Thai beef, cut into thin strips (see page xx)
3 tomatoes, thickly sliced, to serve

for the dressing:
50 ml/2 fl oz sherry vinegar
200 ml/7 fl oz extra virgin olive oil
sea salt flakes, freshly ground black pepper
2 tsp fresh root horseradish, grated

Cut the onion in half and then into very thin slices. Put the rocket into a bowl, add the onion and basil and toss together. Put the dressing ingredients into a jar and shake until blended. Add the beef and tomatoes, drizzle the dressing over the salad and toss everything together.

Top tip:

Horseradish is a pungent root, rich in vitamin C. It is delicious mixed into mash potato.

Harissa with grilled vegetables

Harissa originated in Tunisia although it is now used throughout Morocco and Algeria. It is invariably served with couscous and tagines to add spice and flavour. There are many versions, but this is a particular favourite of mine. To keep the paste, put into a screw-top jar, cover with a thin layer of oil and keep in the fridge.

Serves: 4
Preparation time: 50 minutes
Cooking time: 10 minutes

for the harissa:
1 red pepper, halved and seeded
4 fresh chillies, halved and seeded
olive oil
1 tsp cumin seeds
½ tsp coriander seeds
2 cloves garlic, peeled and finely chopped
1 tbsp paprika
½ tsp cayenne
1 tbsp lemon juice

for the grilled vegetables:
1 fennel bulb, sliced
3 courgettes, trimmed and sliced diagonally
3 carrots, trimmed and sliced diagonally
1 red onion, peeled and sliced

Put the pepper and chillies on to a baking tray, drizzle with oil and rub into the skin. Face the chillies cut side down and put under a hot grill until the skins go black and blister (the pepper will take longer than the chillies). Put the chillies into a plastic bag and leave for 5 minutes (the steam helps to loosen the skin), then peel. Dry fry the cumin and coriander until the seeds start to pop and release their aroma, then crush in a pestle and mortar. Add the garlic, paprika, cayenne and chillies and pound to smooth a paste. Gradually add oil until you have a thick, smooth paste. Add lemon juice and extra cayenne, if you like it really hot.

Put all of the vegetables into a bowl, add 1 tablespoon of harissa paste and toss to coat. Heat a griddle pan until hot, add a little oil, then the vegetables (you may need to do this in batches) and cook for a few minutes until they are tender, but still crunchy and starting to char. Transfer the vegetables to a large bowl, add another 1 tablespoon of harissa (depending on how hot you would like it) and toss everything together.

Top tips:

Harissa is used as a flavouring, sauce or condiment. It is a paste, based on hot red chilli peppers, olive oil and garlic.

Courgettes, otherwise known as zucchini, are miniature marrow, generally available in summer.

Main courses

Lemon and paprika roast chicken with watercress sauce

This is so easy and everyone loves it. I strongly recommend this for a relaxed Sunday lunch with family or friends.

Serves: 4
Preparation time: 20 minutes
Cooking time: about 1 hour 45 minutes (depending on the size of the chicken)

1 medium organic chicken
1 lemon
1 tbsp paprika
sea salt flakes, freshly ground black pepper
550 g/1¼ lb new potatoes
400 g/14 oz fresh watercress
squeeze of lemon juice

Heat the oven to 180°C/350°F/gas mark 4. Trim any excess fat from the chicken (pull out the large piece of fat from inside the body and cut off). Cut the lemon into thin wedges. Rub some of the paprika inside the chicken and stuff with the lemon wedges. Put the chicken on to a wire rack in a roasting tin and sprinkle generously with paprika, salt and pepper. Put into the oven and cook for 40 minutes per kg/2 lb plus 10–15 minutes extra. 40 minutes before the chicken is cooked, add the potatoes to the pan and quickly toss them around to coat with the oil and juices.

Once the chicken is cooked, transfer to a warm platter with the potatoes, then leave to rest for a few of minutes. Spoon out a little of the fat from the pan, put the roasting tray on to a warm hob, add the watercress to the pan and cook for a couple of minutes (not too long, we just want the watercress to wilt, but not cook). Add a squeeze of lemon to the pan of watercress and season to taste. Portion or slice the chicken. Divide the potatoes between four serving plates and top with watercress and slices of chicken. Drizzle over the pan juices, sprinkle with a little extra paprika and serve.

Herb chicken skewers with fresh leaves dressed in oil and lime

This is ideal for cooking outside on the barbeque, so fingers crossed, the weather may be good enough. Serve with bread to mop up the juices.

Serves: 6
Preparation time: 25 minutes (plus 30 minutes marinating time
Cooking time: 5–10 minutes

6 chicken breasts
fresh rosemary sprigs
bunch oregano leaves, roughly chopped
juice of 1 lemon
3 tbsp soy sauce
2 tsp sesame oil
2 cloves garlic, peeled and crushed
2.5 inch/1 cm fresh root ginger, peeled and grated
1 red chilli, seeded and finely sliced
1 tbsp soft brown sugar
300 g/11 oz mixture of leaves, such as watercress, baby spinach, rocket or cos, to serve

for the dressing:
2 tbsp extra virgin olive oil
juice of ½ lime
3 tsp balsamic vinegar

Cut the chicken into thin strips. Thread chicken on to skewers with sprigs of rosemary and oregano. Combine lemon juice, soy sauce, sesame oil, garlic, ginger, chilli and sugar, pour over the chicken, and leave to marinate for 30 minutes. Preheat a griddle pan, grill or barbeque. Cook the chicken for a couple of minutes on each side or until the meat is cooked through, basting with the marinade as the meat cooks. Meanwhile, put the leaves in a bowl. Put the dressing ingredients in a jar and shake to combine, then drizzle over the leaves. Divide the salad between the plates and top with a couple of chicken skewers.

Chicken and citrus fruits with beet and tarragon

This is so easy and it tastes delicious. The oranges and herbs caramelise and go all sticky. As always, buy organic chicken. Beetroot marries well with fruit, especially oranges, apples and redcurrants. This recipe works well because you already have the oven on for the chicken, so the beetroot can be cooked alongside.

If, however, you find yourself on a hot day with some fresh beetroot and you would rather not cook it, simply peel, grate and toss into a salad. Dress with orange juice, balsamic vinegar (this enhances the beet's natural flavour and colour) and a handful of toasted nuts. Always try to buy beetroot with their green leaves attached and choose beets of a similar size so that they cook evenly.

Serves: 6
Preparation time: 20 minutes (plus 30 minutes marinating time)
Cooking time: 35–45 minutes (depending on size of chicken joints)

3 juicy oranges
2 lemons
4 tbsp runny honey
1 tbsp olive oil
large sprigs fresh rosemary
large sprigs fresh tarragon
sea salt flakes, freshly ground black pepper
6 chicken joints
6 garlic cloves, peeled

for the beet:
700 g/1½ lb baby raw beetroot
2 tbsp sherry vinegar
pinch golden caster sugar
zest of 1 orange
handful fresh tarragon, roughly chopped

Preheat the oven to 200°C/400°F/gas mark 6. Squeeze the juice of one of the oranges and one of the lemons into a bowl. Add the honey, oil, half of the herbs, season and mix well. Peel the remaining oranges and lemons. Put the chicken and garlic into a dish, pour over the glaze and toss to coat. Scatter over the sliced fruit. Cover and leave to marinate in the fridge for at least 30 minutes.

Wash the beets thoroughly, then put into a baking tray with a splash of water. Cover tightly with foil and roast for 45 minutes–1 hour, until they are soft when pierced. Remove the beet from the oven, uncover and leave to cool, then peel and cut off their tops and bottom tails. Cut them into quarters or halves and sprinkle with sherry vinegar. Season with sugar, add the orange zest and tarragon and mix everything together.

Transfer the chicken to an ovenproof dish and roast for 35–45 minutes (while you cook the beet), basting occasionally. Five minutes before the end of cooking time, add the rest of the herbs to the pan. Check the chicken is cooked by piercing through the meat with a skewer to see if the middle is cooked and juices run clear. Place a piece of chicken onto each plate, top each with a couple of pieces of fruit and a few herbs and serve with the beetroot.

Moroccan lamb with peach and lemon chutney

A little imagination is required here: we need to picture ourselves in the streets of Morocco with a wonderful aroma coming from the lamb being cooked in a big pan over a little stove. Whenever possible, I grind the spices from whole: they tend to release their oils and flavour as you crush them giving the best possible taste and aroma. Serve this lamb with the chutney, little flat breads and spinach.

Serves: 6
Preparation time: 25 minutes (plus 30 minutes marinating time)
Cooking time: 15 minutes

for the peach and lemon chutney:
6 tsp cumin seeds
3 ripe peaches
50 g/2 oz raisins
2 large onions, peeled and sliced
75 g/3 oz honey
pinch sea salt flakes
1 tsp coriander seeds
juice and zest of 2 lemons
1 tsp paprika
1 cinnamon stick
175 ml/6 fl oz cider vinegar

450 g/1 lb lamb chump steaks, cut into bite-sized pieces
4 tbsp olive oil
pinch salt
2 tsp paprika
1 tsp cinnamon (plus ½ stick, optional)
2 small onions, peeled and cut into thin wedges
paprika, ground cumin, sea salt, to serve
fresh baby spinach and flat breads, to serve

To make the peach and lemon chutney, dry fry the cumin seeds and crush in a pestle and mortar. Put 2 teaspoons of the cumin seeds with all of the other chutney ingredients into a large saucepan and heat gently, stirring for a few minutes. Bring to the boil, then simmer, uncovered, stirring occasionally until all the liquid has evaporated and the mixture is thick. Place the cubed lamb in a dish with half of the oil, salt, 1 teaspoon of paprika, cinnamon (and stick, if using) and 2 more teaspoons of the ground cumin, then mix everything together. Set aside for at least 25 minutes. Heat the remaining oil in a frying pan, add the onions and cook for 20 minutes. Add the lamb and cook for 4 minutes on each side or until lightly charred, turning occasionally. Drizzle the remaining marinade over the meat, add the remaining ground cumin seeds and paprika, and toss together well. Serve with the chutney, little flat breads and extra paprika, cumin and salt to taste.

Thai grilled-beef salad

A hearty salad of meat in a bracing, chilli-lime dressing laced with fresh herbs. This salad is normally served at room temperature and, unlike most savoury Thai dishes, it is not eaten with rice.

Serves: 4
Preparation time: 20 minutes (plus 1 hour marinating time)
Cooking time: 15 minutes

50 ml/2fl oz soy sauce
50 ml/2 fl oz fish sauce (plus extra, to taste)
3 tsp dark soft brown sugar (plus extra, to taste)
450 g/1 lb beef (boneless rib roast)
75 ml/3 fl oz chicken stock
2 spring onions, coarsely chopped
2 shallots, peeled and finely chopped
handful fresh coriander leaves, roughly chopped
1 tsp dried red chilli (plus extra, to taste)
juice of 2 limes
125 g/4 oz lettuce leaves
½ cucumber, peeled, halved and sliced diagonally
5 cherry tomatoes, halved lengthways
a handful fresh mint leaves, roughly chopped

Put the soy sauce, fish sauce and sugar into a glass bowl and stir until the sugar has dissolved. Add the beef and marinate for about 1 hour. Heat a griddle pan and cook the beef until it is pink in the middle and dark and moist on the outside, approximately 3 minutes on each side. Leave the beef to rest for a couple of minutes, then thinly slice on a slight angle, and put to one side. Put the chicken stock in a small saucepan and bring to a gentle boil. Add the beef and warm it in the stock for 1 minute, turning occasionally. Transfer the beef to a bowl. Add the onions, shallots, coriander, chilli, remaining sugar, remaining fish sauce, and lime juice to the beef, and toss well. Taste the dressing and adjust it to your liking with additional fresh fish sauce, lime juice, sugar, or chillies. Arrange the lettuce leaves on a serving platter. With a slotted spoon, transfer the beef to the platter, mounding it on the lettuce. Drizzle over the sauce from the pan and scatter over the cucumber, tomatoes and mint. Serve at room temperature.

Japanese style tuna with sweet and hot cucumber

Wasabi is excellent for really getting those taste buds tingling. But be careful – wasabi is Japanese horseradish and it has real attitude! You only need a little to get the real effect. Pickled ginger is another useful store cupboard ingredient. Make sure that you choose pickled ginger that is a subtle natural colour and not a vivid bright pink caused by food colouring.

Serves: 4 (or 6, as a starter)
Preparation time: 20 minutes plus 4 hours marinating time
Cooking time: about 10 minutes

4 x 175 g/6 oz tuna steaks (about 2.5 cm/1 inch thick)

for the tuna marinade:
4 tbsp sake
2 tbsp soy sauce
1 tsp chilli oil
juice of ½ lemon
1 tbsp vegetable oil

for the sweet and hot cucumber:
½ cucumber
½ red onion, peeled and cut into very thin wedges
1 red chilli, seeded and finely chopped
1 tsp golden caster sugar
1 tbsp warm water
juice of ½ lime
2 tbsp rice wine vinegar
wasabi and pickled ginger, to serve

Put all of the ingredients for the marinade into a bowl, and mix together. Add the tuna, cover and refrigerate for at least 4 hours. Cut the cucumber in half lengthways, scoop out the seeds and very thinly slice each half. Put the cucumber into a bowl, finely chop the red onion, then add to the cucumber with the chilli. Put the sugar and water into a bowl and mix until dissolved. Add the lemon juice and rice wine vinegar and mix together. Pour the dressing over the cucumber and mix everything together. Heat a griddle pan and cook the tuna steaks for 2–4 minutes on each side, or until cooked on the outside and rare in the middle. Spoon the cucumber on to plates, slice the tuna and arrange on top. Serve with a little pickled ginger and a little wasabi.

Top tips:

Sake is a fine distilled rice spirit normally drunk lukewarm.

Wasabi is a Japanese plant and its roots yield one of the hottest spices. The bright green flesh of the root is grated and used fresh or is dried and ground into a paste, or dried as a powder.

Sashimi salmon, sushi rice and toasted nori

This is by far my favourite way of eating. I love to start supper with a fresh green salad lightly dressed with oil and lemon and then follow with fresh fish very lightly cooked and served with nori seaweed and rice.

Serves: 4
Preparation time: 25 minutes (plus 1–2 hours marinating time)
Cooking time: 10 minutes (plus 15 minutes standing time)

450 g/1 lb sashimi salmon
2 tsp sesame oil
2 tsp fresh root ginger, peeled and grated
4 tbsp soy sauce
2 tbsp mirin
2 tbsp lime juice
1 tbsp fresh parsley, roughly chopped
450 ml/¾ pint water
225 g/8 oz Japanese sushi rice
3 sheets nori seaweed
pickled ginger
wasabi, soy sauce and pickled ginger, to serve

Brush the salmon with sesame oil. Heat a frying pan over a high heat. In the frying pan, cook the salmon for 5 seconds on each side, then put to one side. Put the ginger, soy, mirin, lime juice and parsley in a shallow dish. Put the salmon in the marinade, then cover and refrigerate for 1–2 hours, turning occasionally. Slice the salmon thinly. Put the water and rice into a large pan. Bring to the boil, cover and simmer for 10 minutes. Leave to stand (still covered) for 15 minutes. Put half of the rice on to a piece of baking paper, rest on a sushi mat and roll the rice into a long sausage. Cut into 2 cm/1 inch thick pieces. Repeat with the rest of the rice. Toast the nori seaweed, by passing it very quickly under a hot grill or over a gas flame. Cut the seaweed into small squares and place a few on each plate. Top with rice, pickled ginger and salmon. Serve with wasabi, soy sauce and extra pickled ginger.

Top tips:

Sushi and sashimi are the two superlative Japanese raw fish dishes.

Seaweed is a good source of iodine.

Mirin is a very thick and sweet rice wine that is never drunk. It gives a very subtle sweet flavour. Good substitutes are sweet sherry or sake with a little sugar.

Salmon with herb crust and red wine sauce, served with broccoli and Puy lentils

Timing is important with this dish, you need to cook the lentils while the fish is cooking so that they are ready at the same time. The lentils should not be left for too long once they are cooked as they start to go mushy.

Serves: 6
Preparation time: 30 minutes
Cooking time: 20 minutes

6 salmon fillets, skinned

for the marinade:
2 tbsp tarragon, roughly chopped (reserve the stems)
2 tbsp parsley, roughly chopped (reserve the stems)
bunch fresh chives, finely chopped
3 tbsp rock salt
1 tbsp golden caster sugar
zest of 1 lime

for the lentils:
350 g/12 oz Puy lentils, rinsed
2 carrots, peeled and diced
2 sticks celery
1 small onion, peeled and finely chopped
2 cloves garlic, peeled and finely chopped
4 sprigs thyme
½ tsp rock salt

for the sauce:
300 ml/10 fl oz red wine
100 ml/3½ fl oz port
50 ml/2 fl oz red wine vinegar
2 shallots, peeled and finely chopped
50 g/2 oz unsalted butter
fresh broccoli, steamed, to serve

Put the tarragon, parsley, chives, salt, sugar and zest into a bowl and mix together. Spread the marinade on to both sides of the salmon, cover and marinade for at least 1 hour. Preheat the oven to 180°C/350°F/gas mark 4. Put the lentils into a saucepan with the carrots, celery, onions, garlic, thyme and rock salt, cover with cold water, bring to a simmer, cover and cook for 15 minutes. Remove from the heat and leave to stand, covered, for 5 minutes. Meanwhile, brush the herb and salt marinade off the salmon. Heat a heavy griddle pan until very hot and sear the fillets lightly, approximately 1 minute on each side. Transfer to a baking sheet and cook in the oven for 7–10 minutes.

To make the sauce; put the red wine, port, red wine vinegar, shallots and herb stems into a saucepan, bring to the boil and reduce to approximately 100 ml/ 3½ fl oz. Strain into a clean saucepan, bring back to the boil, then reduce the heat. Gradually whisk the butter into the sauce and season well.

Spoon the lentils on to warm plates, top with the salmon and drizzle with the sauce. Serve with freshly steamed broccoli.

Cod with chillies and lemon, served with spinach in sesame-seed dressing

I love suppers like this: they are quick, simple and healthy. With all of the recipes in this section, serve extra vegetables wherever possible to bulk up your vitamin and mineral intake.

Serves: 4
Preparation time: 15 minutes
Cooking time: 10 minutes

4 cod steaks, at least 250 g/9 oz each in weight
2 tbsp olive oil
handful fresh oregano leaves
1 fresh red chilli, seeded and finely chopped
sea salt flakes, freshly ground black pepper
2 lemons, cut into chunks
pinch golden caster sugar
2 bunches spinach

for the sesame seed dressing:
50 g/2 oz white sesame seeds
½ tsp sugar
1½ tbsp soy sauce
2 tbsp dashi

Preheat the oven to 220°C/425°F/gas mark 7. Rinse the cod and dry with kitchen paper. Put the oil, herbs and chilli into a small bowl and mix everything together. Drizzle the oil mixture over the fish, using your hands to really rub the herbs and chilli into the fish, and season well. Put a solid roasting tray into the oven and heat until really hot. Put the fish on to the tray, add the lemons and sprinkle with a little sugar. Cook for 10 minutes.

Meanwhile, make the dressing; dry roast the sesame seeds in a frying pan over a medium heat, shaking the pan constantly. When the seeds begin to pop, remove from the heat. Reserve 1 teaspoon and, using a coffee grinder, grind the remaining seeds until smooth. Add the other ingredients and mix well. Blanch the spinach in boiling water for 40 seconds, drain and gently squeeze out the excess water, then roughly chop. Add the dressing to the spinach, mix together and spoon on to plates. Top with the fish and pop a couple of lemon wedges on the side. Scatter over the reserved sesame seeds and serve.

Top tip:

Use watercress instead of spinach, and macadamias instead of sesame seeds.

Creamy fish curry with cucumber salsa

This curry has an exciting combination of textures and flavours. The creamy sauce is delicious with fish. If you are vegetarian or prefer eating vegetables, add a selection instead of the fish.

Serves: 4
Preparation time: 25 minutes
Cooking time: 25 minutes

1 tbsp olive oil
2 large onions, peeled and finely chopped
2 cloves garlic, peeled and crushed
2 tsp of each sea salt flakes and ground ginger
1 tsp of each ground coriander and turmeric
¼ tsp cumin seeds
¾ tsp ground chilli
400 ml can coconut milk
1 tbsp cornflour
2 tbsp ground almonds
400 g can chopped tomatoes (Ciro, if possible)
300 g/11 oz fresh cod fillet, skinned and cubed
225 g/8 oz raw prawns, peeled, de-veined with tails left on
2 tbsp lime juice
1 tsp golden caster sugar
1 cucumber, peeled, seeded and cubed
bunch fresh coriander, roughly chopped
basmati rice, to serve

Heat the oil in a large heavy-based saucepan, add the onion and garlic and cook until soft. Add the salt, ginger, coriander, turmeric, cumin seeds and chilli, and cook for a few more minutes to really cook the spices, stirring frequently to stop them from burning.

In a separate bowl, make a paste with a little coconut milk and cornflour and mix until smooth. Add the almonds and tomatoes to the saucepan with the cornflour paste and cook for a few minutes. Add the rest of the coconut milk with the chunks of cod and simmer gently until the fish is almost cooked. Add the prawns and a tablespoon of lime juice and cook for a couple of minutes until the prawns are cooked. Mix the rest of the lime juice and sugar together until the sugar has dissolved, then add the cucumber and fresh coriander to make a quick salsa. Serve the curry with freshly cooked basmati rice and the cucumber salsa.

Top tip:

Cod, the world's most abundant saltwater fish, has a lean and white flesh with a delicate flavour. When it is cooked it turns from translucent to white and begins to ooze creamy white juices.

Prawns with Thai flavours

This is for when you want a really quick supper. Serve with noodles and stir-fried greens for a main course or on their own as a starter.

Serves: 4
Preparation time: 10 minutes
Cooking time: 5 minutes

1 tbsp peanut oil
900 g/2 lb cooked prawns
3 shallots, peeled and finely chopped
1 tbsp fresh ginger
2 x 200 g cans water chestnuts, drained and sliced
300 g/11 oz fresh peas
4 kaffir lime leaves
Thai fish sauce, to taste
1 tbsp Thai sweet chilli sauce

Heat the peanut oil in a wok, or large frying pan. Add the remaining ingredients and toss everything together. Cook over a medium heat for 3–4 minutes. Serve.

Top tips:

Kaffir lime leaves are the leaves from a lime tree native to tropical Asia. Crush or slice them to release their strong flavour.

Chinese water chestnut is a tuber, which is cultivated in the East Indies, China and Japan. It is used sliced as a vegetable. In this country it is available in cans.

Roasted peppers with melted cheese

All you need is some fresh crusty bread to help mop up any juices.

Serves: 6
Preparation time: 20 minutes
Cooking time: 1 hour 5 minutes

2 red peppers
2 orange peppers
2 cloves garlic, peeled and chopped
250 g/9 oz pomodorino tomatoes, roughly chopped
2 tbsp extra virgin olive oil, plus extra for drizzling
125 g/4 oz handful olives
150 g/5 oz mozzarella or feta cheese
handful fresh basil and parsley, roughly chopped

Preheat oven to 190°C/375°F/gas mark 5. Quarter and seed the peppers and put into a roasting dish, skin side down. Roast for 30 minutes. Mix together the garlic, tomatoes and olive oil, and season. Spoon a little of this mixture into each pepper. Bake for another 30 minutes, until the peppers are really soft. Cut the cheese into strips and scatter over the peppers. Sprinkle over the herbs, and return to the oven for a few minutes until the cheese has melted. Season to taste, drizzle with a little oil and serve.

Avocado relish with grilled vegetables and salsa in warm tortillas

I prefer to make this recipe during the summer when the vegetables are at their best. Choose sweet and juicy tomatoes and chillies that are full of heat. Adapt the recipe to suit what is available at the time. If possible, eat this outside, as it is perfect outdoor eating food. Serve the relish, vegetables and salsa in separate bowls with a pile of warm tortillas in the middle.

Serves: 4
Preparation time: 25 minutes (plus 1 hour marinating time)
Cooking time: 15 minutes

2 courgettes, trimmed and sliced
2 red bell peppers, seeded and roughly chopped
1 red onion, peeled and sliced into wedges
1 small squash, peeled and cut into small chunks
125 ml/4 fl oz olive oil
1 clove garlic, peeled and finely chopped
1 bunch fresh oregano
pinch salt

for the tomato salsa:
450 g/1 lb ripe tomatoes, cored and finely chopped
½ red onion, peeled and diced
2 chillies, seeded and finely chopped
handful fresh coriander, roughly chopped
sea salt flakes
cayenne pepper

for the avocado corn relish:
125 ml/4 fl oz olive oil
2 heads corn, kernels removed
sea salt flakes, freshly ground black pepper
1 avocado
1 red pepper, cored and seeded
2 poblano chillies, roasted, peeled and seeded
4 spring onions, thinly sliced
50 ml/2 fl oz red wine vinegar
8 flour tortillas

Put the vegetables in a large bowl with the oil, garlic, oregano and salt. Cover and leave to marinate for up to 1 hour. Make the avocado corn relish; heat half of the oil in a saucepan, add the corn, salt and pepper, and fry for 5 minutes. Transfer the mixture to a large mixing bowl and leave to cool. Stone and skin the avocado then cut the avocado, pepper and roasted chillies into small pieces. Add to the corn, along with the spring onions, red wine vinegar and remaining oil. Mix well and leave for at least 20 minutes to develop the flavours.

To make the salsa, put all of the ingredients into a bowl, mix together and season to taste with salt and cayenne pepper. Cover and leave to marinate.

Heat a griddle pan and cook the vegetables until tender but still with a bite, turning occasionally to avoid charring. To assemble, warm the tortillas in a non-stick frying pan or wrap in foil and warm in a low oven. Divide the vegetables down the centre of each tortilla. Top with avocado relish and drizzle with tomato salsa. Fold the bottom quarter of each tortilla up and roll the side over into a cylinder, then serve.

Top tips:

Tortillas are unleavened Mexican 'pancakes', paper thin and pliable enough to roll. They are usually made with a flour called Masa Harina, which is milled from whole corn kernels that have been steeped in lime, dried and cured. There are wheat tortillas, too. When they are rolled and stuffed they are called tacos. Tortilla chips are simply triangle-shaped tortillas that have been deep fried.

Winter squash are available September to March, although acorn squash is available all year round. Winter squash, especially the orange fleshed variety, are an incomparable source of beta-carotene and most are also rich in iron and potassium.

Thai vegetables

Once you have whizzed the paste, this dish is very quick to make and cook. Spoon any leftover curry paste into a screw-top jar and store in the fridge for up to a week. It is delicious added to curries or soups. If you do not have time to make the paste, there are some very good ones available in shops and supermarkets.

Serves: 4
Preparation time: 20 minutes
Cooking time: 10 minutes

for the curry paste:
5 medium/hot green chillies, seeded and roughly chopped
1½ lemon grass stalks, trimmed and roughly chopped
2 tbsp coriander
1 tsp cumin seeds
2½ cm fresh root ginger, peeled and roughly chopped
4 spring onions, trimmed and roughly chopped
2 cloves garlic, peeled and roughly chopped
1 tsp black peppercorns
½ tsp ground cinnamon
juice and zest of ½ lime

2 tbsp vegetable oil
200 ml/7 fl oz vegetable stock
350 ml/12 fl oz coconut milk
250 g/9 oz fresh mixed vegetables, such as green beans, carrots or corn
4 small round aubergines
2 tbsp soy sauce
1 tsp sugar
½ tsp salt
2 handfuls basil leaves, roughly torn

To make the curry paste, put all of the ingredients in to a food processor and whizz to a smooth purée. Heat the oil in a large saucepan, then quickly stir in 2–3 tablespoons of the curry paste. Cook for 1 minute, then add the vegetable stock and coconut milk, and bring to the boil. Add all the remaining ingredients except the basil and simmer for 8–10 minutes until the vegetables are tender. Stir well, add half of the torn basil leaves and spoon into bowls. Scatter the remaining basil over the top and serve.

Roasted tomato tarts with salsa verde and wild rocket

If you are out to impress, make the pastry circles slightly smaller and serve as a starter. Pile fresh wild rocket and herbs on to the middle of the tarts to give them a real peak. Drizzle a little salsa verde around the tarts (if possible serve on white plates to really show off the vibrant colours).

Serves: 4
Preparation time: 10 minutes
Cooking time: 25 minutes

700 g/1½ lb plum tomatoes
2 cloves garlic, peeled
juice of 2 limes
2 tbsp extra virgin olive oil
sea salt flakes, freshly ground black pepper
1 x 375 g sheet puff pastry
plenty of wild rocket plus extra herbs, to serve

for the salsa verde:
½ cup chervil, roughly chopped
¼ cup chives, roughly chopped
¼ cup parsley, chopped
1 tbsp capers
1 shallot, peeled and finely chopped
zest of 1 lemon
225 ml/8 fl oz extra virgin olive oil
2 anchovy fillets, rinsed and chopped

Preheat the oven to 200°C/400°F/gas mark 6. Put the tomatoes and garlic into a baking dish, pour over the lime juice and oil, season and cook for 40 minutes.

Use a saucer to cut out 4 12.5 cm/5 inch circles from the pastry sheet and pierce with a fork. When the tomatoes have only 15 minutes cooking time left, transfer the pastry to a hot baking tray, and bake in the oven above the tomatoes for 10–15 minutes or until golden and puffy. Remove from the tray and turn over.

To make the salsa verde; put the chopped herbs, capers, shallot and lemon zest in a bowl, add the oil and anchovy fillets, and pound together.

To serve, spoon a little salsa verde on to the pastry circles. Divide the tomatoes between the pastry. Drizzle over a little salsa verde, pile the fresh wild rocket on to the middle and top with a few fresh herbs.

Wild mushroom stew with fresh herb mash

This stew is also delicious served on a bed of polenta or with crispy toasted ciabatta.

Serves: 4
Preparation time: 30 minutes (plus 30 minutes marinating time)
Cooking time: 30 minutes

25 g/1 oz dried porcini slices
250 ml/8 fl oz very hot water
225 g/8 oz field mushrooms
225 g/8 oz chestnut mushrooms
2 tbsp olive oil
2 shallots, peeled and finely chopped
1 clove garlic, peeled and sliced
bunch fresh parsley, roughly chopped
sprigs oregano, leaves removed
2 drops Tabasco
2 tbsp Madeira
1 tbsp softened butter mixed with 1 tsp plain flour
sea salt flakes, freshly ground black pepper

for the herb mash:
900 g/2 lbs potatoes
50 ml/2 fl oz milk
1 tbsp extra virgin olive oil
75 g/3 oz fresh herbs, such as tarragon, mint or parsley, roughly chopped

Put the porcini into a bowl, pour over the warm water, cover and leave to infuse for at least 30 minutes. Make the mash; bring a large pan of water to the boil, add the potatoes, bring back to the boil, reduce the heat and simmer until cooked. Drain, return the potatoes to the pan and heat gently to dry. Heat the milk and oil in a separate saucepan, pour over the potatoes and mash, season well, and add the fresh herbs.

Meanwhile, prepare the mushroom stew; remove the porcini slices from the bowl, squeeze out any juice (putting the stock to one side). Cut the porcini into little pieces, slice the field mushrooms and cut the chestnut mushrooms into chunks. Heat the oil in a frying pan, and fry the onion for a few minutes. Add the porcini and cook for a few minutes. Then add the other mushrooms and cook for a further 5 minutes. Add the garlic, parsley, oregano leaves and Tabasco, and cook for another minute. Add the Madeira and stock and cook until the liquid has reduced by half. Add the butter and flour mixture and stir until the mixture has thickened slightly. Season to taste and serve with the mash.

Top tip:

Mushrooms can be stored for a good few days in the fridge as long as there is good air circulation between them. Always keep mushrooms in paper bags with a few holes punched into them if they are kept in plastic bags they tend to sweat and rot easily. Use as little water as possible when cleaning mushrooms a soft-bristled brush is usually sufficient to remove any dirt.

Aromatic vegetables

This is quite a subtle dish. I love it with Thai jasmine rice and extra chilli.

Serves: 4
Preparation time: 20 minutes
Cooking time: 15–20 minutes

250 ml/9 fl oz vegetable stock
250 ml/9 fl oz coconut milk
1 fresh red chilli, seeded and finely chopped
1 star anise
1 tsp ground coriander
sea salt flakes, freshly ground black pepper
90 g/3½ oz skinned unsalted peanuts, toasted and roughly chopped
300 g/11 oz corn, tomatoes (roughly chopped), fresh peas, courgettes (cut into little strips)
1 tbsp sesame oil
2 garlic cloves, peeled and finely chopped
handful fresh basil leaves

Put the stock, milk, chilli, spices and salt into a pan, bring to the boil and simmer for 10 minutes. Dry fry the peanuts over a slow heat until they start to turn golden, then put to one side. Add the vegetables to the sauce and cook until tender. Remove from the heat and season to taste. Heat the sesame oil in a frying pan, add the garlic, and when it starts to colour and crisp, add the basil leaves and stir-fry briefly until just wilted. Stir the garlic-basil mixture into the vegetables, spoon into warm bowls and scatter the toasted nuts over the top.

Sweet potatoes with yogurt and coriander

I decided it was best to include this recipe among the other quick suppers, but you could eat it for lunch or for a quick snack.

Serves: 4
Preparation time: 15 minutes
Cooking time: 1 hour

4 large sweet potatoes (or 8 small)
a little olive oil
sea salt flakes, freshly ground black pepper
425 g/15 oz fresh spinach
600 ml/20 fl oz yogurt
2 cloves garlic, peeled and crushed
about 1 tbsp lemon juice, to taste
handful fresh coriander leaves, roughly chopped

Preheat the oven to 200°C/400°F/gas mark 6. Make a few slits in the potatoes and rub olive oil all over their skins. Scatter over sea salt flakes and bake for about 1 hour (depending on their size). You need the potatoes to be soft when pierced with a knife. Meanwhile, wash and stem the spinach, wilt very quickly in a hot wok for a few minutes, then chop finely. Add the spinach to the yogurt with the garlic and season with lemon juice, salt and pepper. Pop one or two potatoes on each plate, and slit them open down the middle. Spoon a dollop of the spinach yogurt into each and scatter over fresh coriander.

Roasted vegetables with Puy lentils and spices

I have seen and sampled a combination similar to this in three different restaurants, so I decided to have a go at creating the dish myself. This little number is packed with flavour.

Serves: 6
Preparation time: 30 minutes
Cooking time: 55 minutes

3 small courgettes, sliced diagonally
3 carrots, sliced diagonally
2 red onions, peeled and cut into thin wedges
5 cloves garlic
3 tbsp extra virgin olive oil
sea salt flakes, freshly ground black pepper
450 g/1 lb Puy lentils
1 lemon, cut into chunks
1 bay leaf
2 tbsp ground cumin
1 tsp ground coriander
large pinch (about 7 threads) saffron
½ fresh red chilli, seeded and sliced
1 tsp mustard
handful of each fresh basil, coriander, parsley, roughly chopped
200 g/7 oz fresh spinach
1 tsp tamari

Preheat the oven to 200°C/400°F/gas mark 6. Put the courgettes, carrot slices and onion wedges in to a roasting dish. Add 3 of the garlic cloves. Drizzle with oil, scatter over sea salt and freshly ground black pepper and roast for 30–40 minutes. Put the lentils in a saucepan. Finely slice the remaining garlic and add the lemon, bay leaf, cumin, coriander, saffron, chilli and mustard. Generously cover with cold water, bring to the boil, then reduce the heat and simmer until the lentils are tender, for about 20–40 minutes (depending on how fresh the lentils are). Keep an eye on them to make sure they are cooked and not too pulpy. Add the herbs, spinach and tamari, then simmer for a minute. Serve in warm bowls with the roasted vegetables on top.

Top tip:

Tamari is a premium Japanese wheat-free soy sauce with a sharper taste and stronger aroma than many other soy sauces.

Scallops with mango and shallot

Shallots have a more intense flavour than the sweet onions and at the same time are less hot. There may seem like a lot of shallots in this recipe, but their flavour is more delicate after blanching. The contrast in flavour and texture with the shallots, scallops and mango is just sublime.

Serves: 4
Preparation time: 15 minutes plus 20 minutes standing time
Cooking time: 3–4 minutes

200 g/7 oz shallots, peeled and sliced very thinly
1 tsp sea salt flakes
2 tbsp golden caster sugar
2 tbsp white wine vinegar
20 scallops
250 g/9 oz cherry tomatoes
1 green mango, peeled and thinly sliced
large handful fresh mint leaves
2 tsp fish sauce
1 tbsp lemon juice
2 tbsp peanuts, toasted and roughly chopped

Put the shallots into a bowl, cover with boiling water, and leave for 20 seconds. Drain, rinse under cold water and peel. Place the shallots in a bowl, sprinkle with the salt, toss to combine and stand for 20 minutes. Rinse under cold water, then drain well, pressing with the back of a spoon to remove the excess liquid. Transfer to a bowl, add 1 tablespoon of the sugar and the vinegar, mix well and stand for 10 minutes.

Chargrill the scallops over a high heat for 1 minute each side. Put the scallops, shallots, cherry tomatoes, mango and mint leaves in a bowl and toss to combine. Mix the rest of the sugar, fish sauce and lemon juice in a small bowl and whisk until the sugar dissolves. Pour the dressing over the scallop mixture and toss gently to combine. Spoon the mixture on to serving plates and sprinkle with peanuts.

Top tip:

As scallops are highly perishable they should be served within 24 hours of purchase. There are two parts to a scallop; the muscle is white and the roe is orange. Some people remove the roe, others enjoy the flavour and leave it attached.

Red onions with a crunchy chilli and orange topping

Sometimes, the best suppers are those that are the most basic.

Serves: 4
Preparation time: 30 minutes
Cooking time: 1¼ hours

1.4 kg/3 lb red onions (skin attached)
2 tbsp olive oil, plus extra to serve
50 g/2 oz granary breadcrumbs
1 red chilli, seeded and finely chopped
handful fresh mint, roughly chopped
handful fresh parsley, roughly chopped
zest of 1 orange
handful black olives, stoned and finely sliced

Preheat the oven to 170°C/325°F/gas mark 3. Put the onions into an ovenproof dish and bake for 1¼ hours. Heat the oil in a frying pan, then add the breadcrumbs, chilli and herbs, mixing as you cook. Add the orange zest and black olives and mix together. When the onions are cooked, slice the tops off, squeeze out the insides and divide between four plates. Season and drizzle over a little oil, scatter over the crumbs and serve.

Top tip:

Red onions are one of the mildest types of onions.

6

Something sweet

Something sweet

Sugar is a stimulant (just like coffee and tea) and causes a short energy rush after you have eaten it. Therefore, on the nights when you fancy a dessert, it is sensible to leave at least a couple of hours between eating your dessert and going to bed. Alternatively, have a dessert that contains some fibre as this will help to cushion the sugar swings.

Cardamom risotto with dates or chocolate

If you have had quite a light vegetable-based main course, a carbohydrate rice pudding is just what you need for extra energy. I have spent a lot of time in Rome and have many fond memories of the city. This particular recipe is an adaptation of one of those memories. I remember one evening eating a sweet risotto for dessert and being struck by such a clever idea. As with savoury risotto, always use a proper risotto rice and aim for an end result that is slightly soupy, not mushy.

Serves 4
Preparation time: 10 minutes
Cooking time: about 20 minutes

50 g/2 oz flaked almonds
5 cardamom pods
750 ml/1 ¼ pints milk
25 g/1 oz soft brown sugar (unrefined)
50 g/2 oz butter
125 g/4 oz arborio rice
about 1 tbsp orange blossom honey (or enough to taste)
75 g/3 oz dates, stoned and roughly chopped, or 75 g a good-quality dark chocolate, grated

Dry fry the almonds to toast them until golden. Split open the cardamom pods and take out the seeds, throwing away the green pods. Put the milk, sugar and cardamom seeds into a saucepan and heat to simmering point. Melt the butter in a heavy-based saucepan, add the rice and stir to coat the grains. Add a ladleful of the hot milk and stir well. When the rice has absorbed the milk, add another ladleful, and continue until the rice is *al dente* with a creamy sauce. Serve in bowls with the honey to taste and chopped dates or chocolate.

Little pots of orange custard

Soya milk is low in calories, contains no cholesterol, is packed with disease-fighting compounds and is the ideal substitute to dairy milk.

Serves: 4
Preparation time: 20 minutes
Cooking time: 20 minutes

2 tbsp custard powder
1 tbsp soft brown sugar
600 ml/1 pint soya milk
zest and juice of ½ orange

Mix together the custard powder and sugar with just enough milk to make a smooth paste. Bring the rest of the milk up to boiling point. Add the hot milk to the paste, return to the heat and whisk over a gentle heat until the sauce is thick and smooth. Add orange zest and juice and mix together. Pour into little pots and serve warm or cold.

Creamy lemon parfait

Ice cream (or a frozen dessert) does not need lots of cream to make it rich, creamy and sweet; this little recipe is all the proof you will need. For an ice cream, this recipe is low in fat and still high in calcium.

Serves: 8
Preparation time: 20 minutes (plus freezing time)

150 ml/5 fl oz organic milk
juice of ½ lemon
zest of 4 lemons
125 g/4 oz golden caster sugar
300 g/11 oz low fat (or full fat) organic cream cheese

Put all of the ingredients into a food processor and blend until smooth. Transfer to a container, cover and freeze for 3 hours. Take out of the freezer, put back into the food processor and blend until smooth. Cover, return to the freezer and freeze until firm.

Orange cake

I developed the recipe for this cake when I was eleven and each time I make one I still think it's one of the best cakes I've ever eaten. The sauce is very quick to make.

Serves: 6
Preparation time: 20 minutes
Cooking time: 30 minutes

225 g/8 oz butter
225 g/8 oz golden caster sugar
4 eggs, separated
225 g/8 oz self raising flour
grated zest of 3 oranges, plus extra to decorate
juice of 1 orange

for the sauce:
1½ tsp arrowroot
75 g/3 oz golden sugar
juice of 1 lemon and juice of 1 orange
50 ml/2 fl oz water
knob of butter
3 oranges, very thinly sliced

Preheat the oven to 180°C/350°F/gas mark 4. Grease and base line a 20.5 cm/8 inch loaf tin. Cream the butter and sugar together until light and fluffy. Gradually beat the egg yolks into the mixture, one at a time. Fold the sifted flour into the mixture with the orange zest and juice. Whisk the egg whites until stiff and fold into the cake mixture. Bake for 50–55 minutes. The cake is cooked when a skewer poked into the centre of the cake comes out clean.

Make the sauce; put the arrowroot, sugar, lemon juice, orange juice and water into a saucepan and heat very gently until the sugar has dissolved. Bring to the boil and simmer for a few minutes until the sauce is clear and thick. Add the butter and orange slices and heat through.

Cut the cake into chunks and serve with the sauce and a little fresh lemon or orange zest on top.

Top tip:

Arrowroot is available from most good supermarkets and is great for thickening clear sauces.

Espresso brûlée

It is best to make the custard the night before to give it plenty of time to chill and set. Eat this pudding a good few hours before you go to bed.

Serves: 6
Preparation time: 30 minutes (plus chilling time)
Cooking time: 15 minutes

250 ml/9 fl oz double cream
250 ml/9 fl oz whole milk
1 tbsp espresso coffee powder
4 egg yolks
50 g/2 oz golden caster sugar
2 tsp cornflour
125 g/4 oz golden caster or granulated sugar, for the topping

for the toffee sauce:
40 g/1½ oz butter
75 g/3 oz soft brown sugar
2 drops vanilla extract
100 ml/3 fl oz double cream

Put the cream, milk and espresso coffee into a saucepan and heat gently to just below simmering point. Put the egg yolks into a bowl with the sugar and cornflour, then whisk until thick and creamy. Gradually pour the hot cream into the egg mixture, whisking continuously. Pour the custard back into the saucepan and cook gently until the mixture is thick and smooth (do not over-heat at this point). Pour the custard into six ramekins (or coffee cups), cover and leave to cool. Refrigerate overnight.

To make the crisp caramel topping; put a couple of drops of water into a saucepan, add the golden caster sugar and heat very gently. Once the sugar has dissolved it will turn into a caramel; pour this over the custards to form a thin layer. The caramel will turn crisp as it cools.

Make the toffee sauce; put the butter and sugar into a pan and heat gently until melted. Add the vanilla extract and cream and bring up to simmering point. Allow to bubble until the sauce is smooth and thick.

To serve, put a little pot of brûlée on to a plate with a little pot of toffee sauce alongside.

Brown sugar and hazelnut meringues

An excellent dessert for serving in the garden, ideal for when you are entertaining lots of friends or just a couple.

Makes: 14 meringues
Preparation time: 20 minutes
Cooking time: 1½ hours

50 g/2 oz hazelnuts (with skin on), roughly chopped
125 g/4 oz golden caster sugar
125 g/4 oz light soft brown sugar
4 egg whites
150 ml/5 fl oz thick and creamy yogurt
drop vanilla extract
fresh mint leaves, to decorate

for the berry sauce:
450 g/1 lb frozen mixed berries, thawed
golden icing sugar

Preheat the oven to 110°C/225°F/gas mark 1. Put the hazelnuts in a frying pan and dry fry until toasted and golden all over, then leave to cool. Line two baking trays with bakewell paper. Mix the two sugars together in a bowl until they are completely mixed together. Put the egg whites into a clean bowl and whisk with an electric whisk until stiff. Add half of the sugar and whisk again until the mixture is stiff and shiny. Add the remaining sugar and whisk the mixture quickly (it is important to whisk quickly to prevent the egg whites from collapsing). Put tablespoonfuls of the meringue mixture on to the trays, leaving a little space between each one. Put the trays into the oven and bake for 1½ hours. Turn the oven off and leave the meringues to cool before peeling off the paper.

Make the sauce; put half of the berries into a saucepan and heat gently. Mash the fruits to a purée and sift until smooth. Add the remaining whole fruits to the purée and heat gently. Sweeten to taste with the golden icing sugar. Serve the meringues with a dollop of vanilla yogurt and berry sauce. Scatter over a few fresh mint leaves and serve.

Top tips:

Layer the meringues in an airtight container with sheets of bakewell paper between each layer. Make sure the container is completely airtight. Freeze for up to 3 months. When you come to eat the meringues, take a bag of frozen fruits out of the freezer at the same time to make a sauce.

It is vitally important that you use unrefined sugar: it transforms a normal egg white mixture into meringues with a fudgey flavour and slightly soft honeycomb centre.

Bakewell paper may be more expensive than greaseproof paper, but nothing ever sticks to it!

Orange and passion fruit sorbet

Having spent three years as a development chef for a company that produces ice creams and sorbets, I am rather fussy when it comes to eating fruit sorbets or sherbets. The most important thing in my mind when you are making sorbets is to use plenty of fresh juice and very little, if any, water. This way you are guaranteed a good flavour (and more chance of vitamins and minerals) in every mouthful. The sugar is necessary to help give the sorbet a soft and creamy texture.

Serves: 4
Preparation time: 20 minutes (plus freezing time)
Cooking time: 5 minutes

2 kg/4½ lb oranges
250 g/8 oz golden caster sugar
10 passion fruit

Scoop out the inside of the oranges and strain the juice, pressing the pulp firmly against the sieve. Put the juice in a pan with the sugar and heat gently to dissolve. Leave to cool. Cut 9 of the passion fruit in half, scoop the flesh out of the middle into a jug and reserve the shells. Strain the juice, pressing the pulp against the sieve, into a bowl. Mix the passion fruit juice into the orange mixture. Freeze in an ice cream machine. Alternatively, transfer to a freeze-proof container, cover and freeze for 2 hours. Remove from the freezer, use a fork or electric whisk to bash it up and break down the ice crystals, return to the freezer and leave for 2 more hours, then repeat the process. Return the sorbet to the freezer until it hardens (it will take about 2–3 hours).

Scoop the sorbet into the reserved passion fruit shells, cut the remaining passion fruit in half and drizzle a little of its juice over each sorbet.

Index

Figures in bold indicate main references.

acid-forming foods 7, 9, 12, 21
additives 2, 3, 5, 34
alcohol 9, 14, 15, 16, 20
alfalfa sprouts 30
Alfalfa sprouts with spicy tomato salsa and houmous 117
alkaline-forming foods 7, 8, 9, 21
allergies 5
almonds 62
Granola 53
Let's go nutty 42
Muesli – Bircher style 51
Soy nuts 122
Spiced muesli 52
amino acids 3, 4, 6, 7, 12, 23
anchovies
Fresh tuna Niçoise 87
Tapenade toasts 129
antioxidants 4, 16, 21, 37, 62
Antipasto of peppers 135
apples 32
Apple spread for malt loaf 68
Apple and toasted hazelnut flapjacks 71
Berry and apple sundae 67
Berry soup 46
Buttermilk oats with fruit and nuts 54
Carrot-apple zinger 43
Cold fruit compôte 49
Granola 53
Green juice 44
Muesli – Bircher style 51
Spiced apple sauce 45
apricots 32, 62
Cold fruit compôte 49
Couscous with fruits and spices 104
Granola 53
Hot fruit compôte with vanilla yogurt 47
Nutty fruity slice 71
Spiced muesli 52
Warm apricots with ginger 52
Aromatic vegetables 156
artichokes 119
asparagus 31
Baby asparagus 137
Poached free-range eggs served with fresh spinach 54
Roasted asparagus with a lime vinaigrette 89
aubergines 119
Roasted aubergine and bean dip 125
Roasted aubergine, tomatoes and pesto in a baguette 115
Thai vegetables 153
Warm vegetable salad 86
avocados 14, 119
Avocado relish with grilled vegetables and salsa in warm tortillas 152
Avocado with yogurt, lime and red onions 116
Chicken with avocado 102
Guacamole 124
Open avocado and tomato sandwiches 131
Spicy guacamole with roasted vegetables 117
Vegetarian sushi 105

Baby asparagus 137
Baby spinach with crispy bacon and soft creamy eggs 94
Baby spinach with mushrooms, pine nuts and blue cheese 96
bacon
Baby spinach with crispy bacon and soft creamy eggs 94
Bacon and glazed chicken livers 88
Hot bacon bites 127
bananas 33
Banana and bran muffins 57
Banana, fig and honey cake 133
Bananas with cinnamon on toast 50
Dates with cream cheese and banana 72
Hot bananas 66
Hot oranges with crushed cardamom 66
Kiwi, banana and strawberry smoothie 39
Paradise punch 42
Barbecued corn with chilli oil 136
basil 34
Basil aïoli, tomatoes, mozzarella and rocket in granary toast 116
Cannelini beans with tomatoes and basil 91
Spaghetti with marinated tomatoes, fresh basil and garlic crumbs 108
Tomatoes with fresh basil and Parmesan 94
Watercress with red chilli and basil 99
Basil aïoli, tomatoes, mozzarella and rocket in granary toast 116
bay leaves: Chickpeas and sun-blush tomatoes with fresh herb dressing 99
beans 7, 9, 12, 21, **28**
Bean purée with fresh mint and spinach 72
Broad beans with ham or cheese 100
Cannelini beans with tomatoes and basil 91
Fresh tuna Niçoise 87
Roasted aubergine and bean dip 125
Thai vegetables 153
beef 25
Beef with rocket and balsamic vinegar 102
Rocket and beef salad with a horseradish dressing 139
Thai grilled-beef salad 145
beetroot 31
Beetroot with horseradish 74
Beetroot and yogurt 125
Chicken and citrus fruits with beet and tarragon 143
Fresh herb and lemon juice 123
Spicy vegetable juice cocktail 44
berries 119
Berry and apple sundae 67
Berry soup 46
Berry toasts 50
Brown sugar and hazelnut meringues 165
Chocolate and berry cake 133
Fast berry ice cream 132
frozen 34
Intense berry fool 68
Warm berry and currant salad 65
biscuits: Frozen ice cream crunch with crushed raspberries 70
blackberries
Berry and apple sundae 67
Intense berry fool 68
Raspberry and blackberry purée 48
blackcurrants 33
Blackcurrant purée with yogurt 49
blood sugar 2, 5, 11, 15, 20, 37, 61
blueberries 33
Berry and apple sundae 67
Berry soup 46
Blueberry buttermilk pancakes 48
Buttermilk oats with fruit and nuts 54
Lemon and orange cups with crushed blueberries 69
Spiced muesli 52
Warm berry and currant salad 65
bran: Banana and bran muffins 57
brazil nuts
Chocolate and berry cake 133
Nutty fruity slice 71
Soy nuts 122
bread 8, 20, 21
Alfalfa sprouts with spicy tomato salsa and houmous 117
Avocado with yogurt, lime and red onions 116
Baby spinach with crispy bacon and soft creamy eggs 94
Bananas with cinnamon 50
Basil aïoli, tomatoes, mozzarella and rocket in granary toast 116
Bean purée with fresh mint and spinach 72
Beetroot with horseradish 74

Berry toasts 50
Chicken with avocado 102
Chilled gazpacho with spicy cayenne croûtons 79
Cottage cheese with pineapple 74
Crispy bread with plums on top 64
Dates with cream cheese and banana 72
Egg mayo with cress 73
frozen 34
Herby tomatoes 73
Homemade sea salt and rosemary flat breads 103
Open avocado and tomato sandwiches 131
Roasted aubergine, tomatoes and pesto in a baguette 115
Roasted pepper focaccia 115
Spaghetti with marinated tomatoes, fresh basil and garlic crumbs 108
Spicy guacamole with roasted vegetables 117
Tapenade toasts 127
toppings 119
breakfast, eating 37
British Food Calendar 2, 25, 26-7
broad beans 34
Broad bean salad with ham or cheese 100
broccoli: Salmon with herb crust and red wine sauce, served with broccoli and Puy lentils 148
brose: Buttermilk oats with fruit and nuts 54
Brown sugar and hazelnut meringues 165
BSE (bovine spongiform encephalopathy) 5
Butter bean paté 126
buttermilk
Blueberry buttermilk pancakes 48
Buttermilk oats with fruit and nuts 54

cabbages 32
Green juice 44
caffeine 16, 20
cakes
Banana, fig and honey cake 133
Chocolate and berry cake 133
Orange cake 163
calcium 15, 16
cancer 1, 2, 7, 9, 16, 23, 37
cannellini beans
Cannelini beans with tomatoes and basil 91
Roasted aubergine and bean dip 125
capers
Pasta with lemon, rocket and chilli 109
Tapenade toasts 127
Caramelised leek puff 108
carbohydrates 1, 2, 6-11, 19, 20, 21, 23, 77
cardamom
Cardamom risotto with dates or chocolate 161
Hot oranges with crushed cardamom 66
carrots 32
Carrot soup with honey and ginger 80
Carrot with nuts and raisins in a tangy orange dressing 100
Carrot-apple zinger 43
Fresh herb and lemon juice 123
New potato salad 90
Roasted pepper and vegetable soup 83
Roasted vegetables with Puy lentils and spices 157
Spicy vegetable juice cocktail 44
Thai vegetables 153
cashew nuts 119
Granola 53
Muesli – Bircher style 51
Spiced muesli 52
celery 30
Carrot soup with honey and ginger 80
New potato salad 90
Roasted pepper and vegetable soup 83
Spicy vegetable juice cocktail 44
Watercress and potato soup 78
cell metabolism 3
chard: Green juice 44
cheese 7, 21, 30, **30**
Baby spinach with mushrooms, pine nuts and blue cheese 96
British Food Calendar 26, 27
Broad bean salad with ham or cheese 100
Caramelised leek puff 108
Cheese and mint 126
Pan-fried fresh goat's cheese with roast tomatoes and garlic 113
Pepper salad 98
Roasted peppers with melted cheese 151
Tomato salad with cucumbers, feta cheese, oregano and mint 97
cherries 33
Chicken with cherries 114
chewing food 6
chicken 21, 25
Bacon and glazed chicken livers 88
Chicken with avocado 102
Chicken with cherries 114
Chicken and citrus fruits with beet and tarragon 143
Griddled chicken 112
Herb chicken skewers with fresh leaves dressed in oil and lime 142
Lemon and paprika roast chicken with watercress sauce 141
Sweet and sour glazed chicken 113
chickpeas
Bean purée with fresh mint and spinach 72
Chickpeas and sun-blush tomatoes with fresh herb dressing 99
Houmous 123
Italian chickpea soup with pesto 85
chicory 32
Spinach with satsumas and a ginger vinaigrette 95
Chilled gazpacho with spicy cayenne croûtons 79
Chilli peanuts 121
chillies 31
Barbecued corn with chilli oil 136
Cod with chillies and lemon, served with spinach in sesame-seed dressing 149
Guacamole 124
Harissa with grilled vegetables 140
Hot chilli olives 120
Jasmine rice pilaff with chunky tomato salsa 106
Pasta with lemon, rocket and chilli 109
Red onions with a crunchy chilli and orange topping 159
Spicy guacamole with roasted vegetables 117
Spicy peanut sauce with vegetables and toasts 126
Thai vegetables 153
Tiger prawns with chilli and garlic 112
Watercress with red chilli and basil 99
chives 34
Tomatoes with chives 132
chocolate
Cardamom risotto with dates or chocolate 161
Chocolate and berry cake 133
chutney: peach and lemon 144
ciabatta 119
Spicy guacamole with roasted vegetables 117
cinnamon
Apple spread for malt loaf 68
Bananas with cinnamon 50
citrus fruits 7
coconut
Granola 53
Spiced muesli 52
coconut milk 28
Mango and coconut smoothie 38
Pineapple and coconut milk 40
Thai sweetcorn soup with coconut 84
cod
Cod, with chillies and lemon, served with spinach in sesame-seed dressing 149
Creamy fish curry with cucumber salsa 150
coffee 1, 7, 14, 20
Espresso brûlée 164
compôtes
Cold fruit compôte 49
Hot fruit compôte with vanilla yogurt 47
Rhubarb compôte 45
Rhubarb and ginger compôte 64
coriander 34
Fresh herb and lemon juice 123
Sweet potatoes with yogurt and coriander 156
corn
Barbecued corn with chilli oil 136
Spicy popcorn 121
Thai vegetables 153
Cottage cheese with pineapple 74
courgettes
Aromatic vegetables 156
Avocado relish with grilled vegetables and salsa in warm tortillas 152
Roasted vegetables with Puy lentils and spices 157
Warm vegetable salad 86
couscous 8
Couscous with fruits and spices 104
Couscous with grilled tomatoes and red onions 88-9
cranberries 33
Cranberry and orange 41
Nutty fruity slice 71
Spiced muesli 52
Wild rice salad with tangerines and pine nuts 101
cream cheese
Beetroot with horseradish 74
Creamy lemon parfait 162
Dates with cream cheese and banana 72
Creamy fish curry with cucumber salsa 150
Creamy lemon parfait 162
Creamy smoked mackerel 110
cress
Egg mayo with cress 73
Fresh green salad with Parmesan crisps 139
Crispy bread with plums on top 64
cucumbers 119
Beetroot and yogurt 125
Chilled gazpacho with spicy cayenne croûtons 79
Creamy fish curry with cucumber salsa 150
Green juice 44
Japanese style tuna with sweet and hot cucumber 146
Salmon with lime and yogurt 131
Spicy vegetable juice cocktail 44
Thai grilled-beef salad 145
Tiger prawns with chilli and garlic 112
Tomato salad with cucumbers, feta cheese, oregano and mint 97
Vegetarian sushi 105
curd cheese 119
currants
Couscous with fruits and spices 104
Warm berry and currant salad 65
Wild rice salad with tangerines and pine nuts 101

dairy foods 21
dates 62
Cardamom risotto with dates or chocolate 161
Dates with cream cheese and banana 72
Granola 53
Let's go nutty 42
detoxification 37
diet
and activity levels 18-19
the benefits of a traditional diet 2
the challenges of a modern diet 2
crash dieting 6
digestion 3, 5, 6-9, 21, 77, 135
dips
Beetroot and yogurt 125
Cheese and mint 126

Guacamole 124
Roasted aubergine and bean dip 125
dried fruit 62
Granola 53
Nutty fruity slice 71
drinks 38-44

eating habits 5
eggs 7, 21, 135
Baby spinach with crispy bacon and soft creamy eggs 94
Egg mayo with cress 73
Espresso brûlée 164
Omelettes 55
Poached free-range eggs served with fresh spinach 54
Scrambled eggs with herbs and smoked salmon 56
Soft eggs with tomatoes and watercress 137
electrolytes 3
endives: Chicken with avocado 102
energy, sources of 10-19
enzymes 3, 4, 6, 7, 12, 15, 16, 24, 37
Espresso brûlée 164
essential amino acids 12
essential fatty acids 11, 23
exercise 16, 19, 21

Fast berry ice cream 132
fat 1, 2, 6, 7, 9, **13-14**, 19
saturated 7, 9, 13, 20
unsaturated 13, 14, 62
fatty acids 6, 119
fennel 32
Fennel soup with lemon oil 82
Fresh herb and lemon juice 123
Pear, fennel and walnut salad 98
Watercress, orange and fennel 93
fertilisers 23, 24
feta cheese
Roasted peppers with melted cheese 151
Tomato salad with cucumbers, feta cheese, oregano and mint 97
fibre 7, 8, 11, **12**, 20, 21, 23, 37
figs 62
Banana, fig and honey cake 133
Let's go nutty 42
filo pastry 34
fish 20, 21
British Food Calendar 26, 27
see also cod; herrings; mackerel; salmon
flapjacks: Apple and toasted hazelnut flapjacks 71
focaccia: Roasted pepper focaccia 115
food combining 8-9
freezer 34
French beans: Italian chickpea soup with pesto 85
Fresh green salad with Parmesan crisps 139
Fresh herb and lemon juice 123
Fresh leaves with tomatoes and goat's cheese 138
Fresh tuna Niçoise 87
frisée: Spinach with satsumas and a ginger vinaigrette 95
Frozen ice cream crunch with crushed raspberries 70
fruit 4, 8, 9, 11, 12, 20-21, 24, **32-3**
as breakfast food 37
British Food Calendar 26-7
dried 29
eating separately 8-9, 20
organic 20, 21

game: British Food Calendar 26, 27
garlic 30
Olives with orange, herbs and garlic 120
Olives with rosemary and garlic 120
Pan-fried fresh goat's cheese with roast tomatoes and garlic 113
Soft garlicky peppers 97
Spaghetti with marinated tomatoes, fresh basil and garlic crumbs 108
Tomato soup with garlic and lots of herbs 83
gazpacho: Chilled gazpacho with spicy cayenne croûtons 79
genetically modified foods 5
ginger 30
Carrot soup with honey and ginger 80
Mango and lychees with ginger 69
Melon with ginger 41
Rhubarb and ginger compôte 64
Spinach with satsumas and a ginger vinaigrette 95
Warm apricots with ginger 52
glycerol 6
glycogen 19
goat's cheese 135
Cheese and mint 126
Fresh leaves with tomatoes and goat's cheese 138
Mushrooms with tapenade 136
Pan-fried fresh goat's cheese with roast tomatoes and garlic 113
grains 7, 9, 11, 12, 14, 20, 21, **28**, 63, 119
Granola 53
Frozen ice cream crunch with crushed raspberries 70
grapefruit 33, 62
Pineapple, grapefruit and passion fruit smoothie 39
grapes 32, 62
green beans: Thai vegetables 153
Green juice 44
Griddled chicken 112
Griddled sweet potato 128
guacamole 119
Guacamole 124
Spicy guacamole with roasted vegetables 117

ham: Broad bean salad with ham or cheese 100
Harissa with grilled vegetables 140
hazelnuts
Apple and toasted hazelnut flapjacks 71
Berry and apple sundae 67
Brown sugar and hazelnut meringues 165
Buttermilk oats with fruit and nuts 54
Carrot with nuts and raisins in a tangy orange dressing 100
Hot bananas 66
Muesli – Bircher style 51
Tomato and watercress salad with hazelnut dressing 92
heart disease 2, 9, 16, 37
herbs 33-4
British Food Calendar 26, 27
Herb chicken skewers with fresh leaves dressed in oil and lime 142
Olives with orange, herbs and garlic 120
Scrambled eggs with herbs and smoked salmon 56
Tiny pasta with fresh herbs 130
Tomato soup with garlic and lots of herbs 83
Wild mushroom stew with fresh herb mash 153
Herby tomatoes 73
herrings: Marinated herrings 110
Homemade sea salt and rosemary flat breads 103
honey 29, 62
Banana, fig and honey cake 133
Carrot soup with honey and ginger 80
Granola 53
Honeyed pears 65
Muesli – Bircher style 51
Honeyed pears 65
horseradish 31
Beetroot with horseradish 74
Creamy smoked mackerel 110
Rocket and beef salad with a horseradish dressing 139
Hot bacon bites 127
Hot bananas 66
Hot chilli olives 120
Hot fruit compôte with vanilla yogurt 47
Hot oranges with crushed cardamom 66
houmous 30, 119
Alfalfa sprouts with spicy tomato salsa and houmous 117
Houmous 123

ice creams 34, 37, 119
Fast berry ice cream 132
Frozen ice cream crunch with crushed raspberries 70
ingredients 28-34
Intense berry fool 68
iron 15
Italian chickpea soup with pesto 85

Japanese style tuna with sweet and hot cucumber 146
Jasmine rice pilaff with chunky tomato salsa 106
juices 21, 37, 38, 62

kale 31
Green juice 44
Kippers with parsley and pepper 58
kiwi fruit 33, 62
Kiwi, banana and strawberry smoothie 39
Kiwi mania 43

lamb 25
Moroccan lamb with peach and lemon chutney 144
lavender: Oranges with lavender 46
leeks 32
Caramelised leek puff 108
Fennel soup with lemon oil 82
Italian chickpea soup with pesto 85
Roasted pepper and vegetable soup 83
lemon grass 31
lemons 33
Creamy lemon parfait 162
Fennel soup with lemon oil 82
Lemon and orange cups with crushed blueberries 69
Lemon and paprika roast chicken with watercress sauce 141
Moroccan lamb with peach and lemon chutney 144
Pasta with lemon, rocket and chilli 109
lentils 9, 12, 21
Lentils with herbs and balsamic vinegar 101
Roasted vegetables with Puy lentils and spices 157
Salmon with herb crust and red wine sauce, served with broccoli and Puy lentils 148
Let's go nutty 42
lettuce
Chicken with avocado 102
Cottage cheese with pineapple 74
Fresh leaves with tomatoes and goat's cheese 138
Herb chicken skewers with fresh leaves dressed in oil and lime 142
Marinated herrings 110
Pea and lettuce soup 81
Warm vegetable salad 86
limes 33
Avocado with yogurt, lime and red onions 116
Cod, with chillies and lemon, served with spinach in sesame-seed dressing 149
Herb chicken skewers with fresh leaves dressed in oil and lime 142
Moroccan lamb with peach and lemon chutney 144
Papaya with passion fruit and lime 43
Roasted asparagus with a lime vinaigrette 89
Salmon with lime and yogurt 131
linseeds 29
liqueurs
Fast berry ice cream 132
Intense berry fool 68
Little pots of orange custard 162
liver, the 9
lunches, eating 77

lychees: Mango and lychees with ginger 69

mackerel: Creamy smoked mackerel 110
magnesium 15, 16
mangoes 33, 62
Mango and coconut smoothie 38
Mango and lychees with ginger 69
Mango purée 49, 70
Paradise punch 42
Scallops with mango and shallot 158
Marinated herrings 110
Marinated salmon 109
marjoram: Chickpeas and sun-blush tomatoes with fresh herb dressing 99
mayonnaise: Egg mayo with cress 73
meat 7, 15, 20, 21
British Food Calendar 26, 27
Oranges and tarragon with cold meats 111
melons 33, 62
Kiwi mania 43
Melon with ginger 41
Melon madness 41
meringues: Brown sugar and hazelnut meringues 165
mid-afternoon snacks, eating 119
mid-morning boosts
eating 61
fruity ideas 62
nutty ideas 62
milk 15, **30**, 38
Creamy lemon parfait 162
Little pots of orange custard 162
minerals 1, 4, 11, **15-16**, 20, 21, 37, 62, 77
mint 33
Bean purée with fresh mint and spinach 72
Cheese and mint 126
Mushrooms with herbs 129
Tomato salad with cucumbers, feta cheese, oregano and mint 97
Moroccan lamb with peach and lemon chutney 144
mozzarella
Basil aïoli, tomatoes, mozzarella and rocket in granary toast 116
Roasted peppers with melted cheese 151
muesli
Muesli – Bircher style 51
Spiced muesli 52
muffins, Banana and bran muffins 57
mung beans 119
mushrooms 119
Baby spinach with mushrooms, pine nuts and blue cheese 96
Mushrooms with herbs 129
Mushrooms with tapenade 136
Sesame mushrooms 138
Warm vegetable salad 86
Wild mushroom stew with fresh herb mash 155

nectarines 62
Warm berry and currant salad 65
New potato salad 90
noodles: Tiger prawns with chilli and garlic 112
nuts 14, 20, **28**, 62
Buttermilk oats with fruit and nuts 54
Nutty fruity slice 71

oats
Apple and toasted hazelnut flapjacks 71
Buttermilk oats with fruit and nuts 54
Granola 53
Muesli – Bircher style 51
Nutty fruity slice 71
Porridge 51
Spiced muesli 52
oils 28-9
olive oil 9, 14
olives 29, 119, 135
black olive spread 119
Hot chilli olives 120
Olives with orange, herbs and garlic 120
Olives with rosemary and garlic 120
Tapenade toasts 127
Tomato puff with pesto and olives 104
Omelettes 55
onions 119
Avocado with yogurt, lime and red onions 116
Couscous with grilled tomatoes and red onions 88-9
Red onions with a crunchy chilli and orange topping 159
Open avocado and tomato sandwiches 131
oranges 33, 62
Carrot with nuts and raisins in a tangy orange dressing 100
Chicken and citrus fruits with beet and tarragon 143
Cranberry and orange 41
Hot oranges with crushed cardamom 66
Lemon and orange cups with crushed blueberries 69
Little pots of orange custard 162
Mango purée 49
Olives with orange, herbs and garlic 120
Orange berry blast 42
Orange cake 163
Orange and passion fruit sorbet 166
Oranges with lavender 46
Oranges and tarragon with cold meats 111
Red onions with a crunchy chilli and orange topping 159
Rhubarb compôte 45
Watercress, orange and fennel 93
oregano: Tomato salad with cucumbers, feta cheese, oregano and mint 97
organic foods 1, 3, 4, 5, 21, **23-4**

Pan-fried fresh goat's cheese with roast tomatoes and garlic 113
pancakes: Blueberry buttermilk pancakes 48
pancetta 135
papaya 33
Papaya with passion fruit and lime 43
Papaya, peach and passion fruit smoothie 40
Paradise punch 42
Parmesan cheese
Fresh green salad with Parmesan crisps 139
Tomatoes with fresh basil and Parmesan 94
parsley 33, 119
Chickpeas and sun-blush tomatoes with fresh herb dressing 99
Fresh herb and lemon juice 123
Kippers with parsley and pepper 58
Mushrooms with herbs 129
Salmon with herb crust and red wine sauce, served with broccoli and Puy lentils 148
passion fruit 33
Orange and passion fruit sorbet 166
Papaya with passion fruit and lime 43
Papaya, peach and passion fruit smoothie 40
Pineapple, grapefruit and passion fruit smoothie 39
pasta 8, 20, **28**
Pasta with lemon, rocket and chilli 109
Tiny pasta with fresh herbs 130
pastry, frozen 34
paté: Butter bean paté 126
peaches 33, 62
Moroccan lamb with peach and lemon chutney 144
Muesli – Bircher style 51
Papaya, peach and passion fruit smoothie 40
Warm berry and currant salad 65
peanuts 62
Aromatic vegetables 156
Chilli peanuts 121
pears 32
Honeyed pears 65
Pear, fennel and walnut salad 98
peas
Aromatic vegetables 156
Italian chickpea soup with pesto 85
Pea and lettuce soup 81
Prawns with Thai flavours 151
pecans
Blueberry buttermilk pancakes 48
Chocolate and berry cake 133
peppers 119, 135
Antipasto of peppers 135
Avocado relish with grilled vegetables and salsa in warm tortillas 152
Fresh herb and lemon juice 123
Harissa with grilled vegetables 140
New potato salad 90
Pepper salad 98
Roasted pepper focaccia 115
Roasted pepper and vegetable soup 83
Roasted peppers with melted cheese 151
Soft garlicky peppers 97
Spicy vegetable juice cocktail 44
Warm vegetable salad 86
pesticides 3, 23, 24
pesto
Italian chickpea soup with pesto 85
Roasted aubergine, tomatoes and pesto in a baguette 115
Tomato puff with pesto and olives 104
petit pois 34
phosphates 23
phosphorus 15
phytochemicals 4, 21
pilaff: Jasmine rice pilaff with chunky tomato salsa 106
pine nuts
Baby spinach with mushrooms, pine nuts and blue cheese 96
Cottage cheese with pineapple 74
Wild rice salad with tangerines and pine nuts 101
pineapples 32
Cottage cheese with pineapple 74
Mango and lychees with ginger 69
Paradise punch 42
Pineapple and coconut milk 40
Pineapple, grapefruit and passion fruit smoothie 39
plums 33
Crispy bread with plums on top 64
Poached free-range eggs served with fresh spinach 54
popcorn: Spicy popcorn 121
pork 25
Porridge 51
potassium 15, 37
potatoes
Fresh tuna Niçoise 87
Lemon and paprika roast chicken with watercress sauce 141
New Potato Salad 90
Soft eggs with tomatoes and watercress 137
Spicy chips 128
Thai sweetcorn soup with coconut 84
Watercress and potato soup 78
Wild mushroom stew with fresh herb mash 153
poultry: British Food Calendar 26, 27
Power Food basics 20-21
prawns
Creamy fish curry with cucumber salsa 150
Prawns with Thai flavours 151
Tiger prawns with chilli and garlic 112
processed foods 1, 2, 20
prosciutto 119, 135
protein 2, 3, 6-9, **12-13**, 15, 16, 19, 20, 38, 62, 77
prunes
Cold fruit compôte 49
Granola 53
Hot bacon bites 127
puff pastry 34
pulses 14, **28**

pumpkin seeds 119
Toasted seeds 122
purées
Bean purée with fresh mint and spinach 72
Blackcurrant purée with yogurt 49
Mango purée 59, 70
Raspberry and blackberry purée 48

radicchio
Chicken with avocado 102
Fresh herb and lemon juice 123
Pear, fennel and walnut salad 98
radishes 31, 135
Spicy vegetable juice cocktail 44
raisins
Buttermilk oats with fruit and nuts 54
Carrot with nuts and raisins in a tangy orange dressing 100
Couscous with fruits and spices 104
Granola 53
Spiced muesli 52
raspberries 62
Berry and apple sundae 67
Berry soup 46
Frozen ice cream crunch with crushed raspberries 70
Intense berry fool 68
Raspberry and blackberry purée 48
Warm berry and currant salad 65
raw foods 1, 3, 4, 6, 8, 21
Red onions with a crunchy chilli and orange topping 159
redcurrants: Warm berry and currant salad 65
rheumatoid arthritis 7
rhubarb
Rhubarb compôte 45
Rhubarb and ginger compôte 64
rice 8, 11, **28**
Jasmine rice pilaff with chunky tomato salsa 106
Sashimi salmon, sushi rice and toasted nori 147
Vegetarian sushi 105
Wild rice salad with tangerines and pine nuts 101
risotto: Cardamom risotto with dates or chocolate 161
Roasted asparagus with a lime vinaigrette 89
Roasted aubergine and bean dip 125
Roasted aubergine, tomatoes and pesto in a baguette 115
Roasted pepper focaccia 115
Roasted pepper and vegetable soup 83
Roasted peppers with melted cheese 151
Roasted tomato tarts with salsa verde and wild rocket 154
Roasted vegetables with Puy lentils and spices 157
rocket
Basil aïoli, tomatoes, mozzarella and rocket in granary toast 116
Beef with rocket and balsamic vinegar 102
Fresh green salad with Parmesan crisps 139
Herb chicken skewers with fresh leaves dressed in oil and lime 142
Marinated herrings 110
Pasta with lemon, rocket and chilli 109
Pear, fennel and walnut salad 98
Roasted pepper focaccia 115
Roasted tomato tarts with salsa verde and wild rocket 154
Rocket and beef salad with a horseradish dressing 139
rosemary 34
Homemade sea salt and rosemary flat breads 103
Olives with rosemary and garlic 120
runner beans: Fresh tuna Niçoise 87

saffron 31
sage 34
Chickpeas and sun-blush tomatoes with fresh herb dressing 99
salad leaves
Bacon and glazed chicken livers 88
Fresh tuna Niçoise 87
Tomato salad with cucumbers, feta cheese, oregano and mint 97
salad leaves, mixed 30
salads 4, 21, 77
salads (cold)
Baby spinach with crispy bacon and soft creamy eggs 94
Baby spinach with mushrooms, pine nuts and blue cheese 96
Beef with rocket and balsamic vinegar 102
Broad bean salad with ham or cheese 100
Cannelini beans with tomatoes and basil 91
Carrot with nuts and raisins in a tangy orange dressing 100
Chicken with avocado 102
Chicken with cherries 114
Chickpeas and sun-blush tomatoes with fresh herb dressing 99
Couscous with fruits and spices 104
Fresh green salad with Parmesan crisps 139
Lentils with herbs and balsamic vinegar 101
Oranges and tarragon with cold meats 111
Pasta with lemon, rocket and chilli 109
Pear, fennel and walnut salad 98
Pepper salad 98
Rocket and beef salad with a horseradish dressing 139
Sardines with watercress 111
Soft garlicky peppers 97
Spaghetti with marinated tomatoes, fresh basil and garlic crumbs 108
Spinach with satsumas and a ginger vinaigrette 95
Tomato salad with cucumbers, feta cheese, oregano and mint 97
Tomato and watercress salad with hazelnut dressing 92
Tomatoes with fresh basil and Parmesan 94
Watercress, orange and fennel 93
Watercress with red chilli and basil 99
Wild rice salad with tangerines and pine nuts 101
salads (warm)
Bacon and glazed chicken livers 88
Couscous with grilled tomatoes and red onions 88-9
Fresh tuna Niçoise 87
New potato salad 90
Roasted asparagus with a lime vinaigrette 89
Thai grilled-beef salad 145
Warm berry and currant salad 65
Warm vegetable salad 86
salmon 119
Marinated salmon 109
Salmon with herb crust and red wine sauce, served with broccoli and Puy lentils 148
Salmon with lime and yogurt 131
Sashimi salmon, sushi rice and toasted nori 147
Scrambled eggs with herbs and smoked salmon 56
salsa
Alfalfa sprouts with spicy tomato salsa and houmous 117
Avocado relish with grilled vegetables and salsa in warm tortillas 152
Creamy fish curry with cucumber salsa 150
Jasmine rice pilaff with chunky tomato salsa 106
Roasted tomato tarts with salsa verde and wild rocket 154
salt 9, 15
Homemade sea salt and rosemary flat breads 103
sandwiches
Alfalfa sprouts with spicy tomato salsa and houmous 117
Avocado with yogurt, lime and red onions 116
Basil aïoli, tomatoes, mozzarella and rocket in granary toast 116
Open avocado and tomato sandwiches 131
Roasted aubergine, tomatoes and pesto in a baguette 115
Roasted pepper focaccia 115
Spicy guacamole with roasted vegetables 117
sardines 119
Sardines with watercress 111
Sashimi salmon, sushi rice and toasted nori 147
satsumas: Spinach with satsumas and a ginger vinaigrette 95
sauces 28
Fresh herb and lemon juice 123
Spiced apple sauce 45
Spicy peanut sauce with vegetables and toasts 126
Tomato sauce for pasta 107
watercress 141
Scallops with mango and shallot 158
scones: Warm tomato scones 129
Scrambled eggs with herbs and smoked salmon 56
sea salt flakes (Maldon) 29
seasonal foods 2, 4, 5, 25-7
seaweed 28
Sashimi salmon, sushi rice and toasted nori 147
Vegetarian sushi 105
seeds 14, 20, **28**
selenium 16, 62
Sesame mushrooms 138
sesame seeds
Cod, with chillies and lemon, served with spinach in sesame-seed dressing 149
Granola 53
Nutty fruity slice 71
shallots: Scallops with mango and shallot 158
smoothies 37
Kiwi, banana and strawberry smoothie 39
Mango and coconut smoothie 38
Papaya, peach and passion fruit smoothie 40
Pineapple, grapefruit and passion fruit smoothie 39
snacks
fruity ideas 62
healthy 60
nutty ideas 62
quick hot 127-30
sodium 15
Soft eggs with tomatoes and watercress 137
Soft garlicky peppers 97
sorbets 34, 119
Orange and passion fruit sorbet 166
soups
Berry soup 46
Carrot soup with honey and ginger 80
Chilled gazpacho with spicy cayenne croûtons 79
Fennel soup with lemon oil 82
Italian chickpea soup with pesto 85
Pea and lettuce soup 81
Roasted pepper and vegetable soup 83
Strawberry soup 47
Thai sweetcorn soup with coconut 84
Tomato soup with garlic and lots of herbs 83
Watercress and potato soup 78
Soy nuts 122
Spaghetti with marinated tomatoes, fresh basil and garlic crumbs 108
Spiced apple sauce 45
Spiced muesli 52
spices 29, 30-31
Spicy chips 128
Spicy guacamole with roasted vegetables 117
Spicy popcorn 121
Spicy vegetable juice cocktail 44
spinach 31
Baby spinach with crispy bacon and soft creamy eggs 94
Baby spinach with mushrooms, pine nuts and blue cheese 96
Bean purée with fresh mint and spinach 72
Cod, with chillies and lemon, served with spinach in sesame-seed dressing 149
Fresh green salad with Parmesan crisps 139
Green juice 44
Herb chicken skewers with fresh leaves dressed

in oil and lime 142
Poached free-range eggs served with fresh spinach 54
Spinach with satsumas and a ginger vinaigrette 95
Sweet potatoes with yogurt and coriander 156
spring onions 119
squash
Avocado relish with grilled vegetables and salsa in warm tortillas 152
Warm vegetable salad 86
strawberries 32, 62
Berry soup 46
Intense berry fool 68
Kiwi, banana and strawberry smoothie 39
Muesli – Bircher style 51
Strawberry soup 47
Warm berry and currant salad 65
stress 1, 6, 7, 15, 16
sugar 1, 2, 7, 10-11, 15, 20, 21, 37
Brown sugar and hazelnut meringues 165
simple 6
unrefined 29
sunflower seeds 62, 119
Granola 53
Nutty fruity slice 71
Spiced muesli 52
Toasted seeds 122
suppers, eating 135
sushi
Sashimi salmon, sushi rice and toasted nori 147
Vegetarian 105
sweet foods, eating 161
sweet potatoes 32
Griddled sweet potato 128
Sweet potatoes with yogurt and coriander 156
Sweet and sour glazed chicken 113
sweetcorn: Thai sweetcorn soup with coconut 84
Swiss Vegetable Bouillon Powder 28

tahini 9, 119
tangerines: Wild rice salad with tangerines and pine nuts 101
tapenade
Mushrooms with tapenade 136
Tapenade toasts 127
tarragon
Chicken and citrus fruits with beet and tarragon 143
Oranges and tarragon with cold meats 111
Salmon with herb crust and red wine sauce, served with broccoli and Puy lentils 148
tea 1, 14, 20, 30, 63
Thai grilled-beef salad 145
Thai sweetcorn soup with coconut 84
Thai vegetables 153
thyme 34
Lentils with herbs and balsamic vinegar 101
Tiger prawns with chilli and garlic 112
Tiny pasta with fresh herbs 130
toast, toppings for (Berry toasts) 50
Toasted seeds 122
tofu 21, 30
tomatoes 32, 119, 135
Alfalfa sprouts with spicy tomato salsa and houmous 117
Aromatic vegetables 156
Basil aïoli, tomatoes, mozzarella and rocket in granary toast 116
Cannelini beans with tomatoes and basil 91
Chicken with avocado 102
Chickpeas and sun-blush tomatoes with fresh herb dressing 99
Chilled gazpacho with spicy cayenne croûtons 79
Couscous with grilled tomatoes and red onions 88-9
Creamy fish curry with cucumber salsa 150
Fresh leaves with tomatoes and goat's cheese 138
Fresh tuna Niçoise 87
Guacamole 124
Herby tomatoes 73
Italian chickpea soup with pesto 85
Jasmine rice pilaff with chunky tomato salsa 106
Lentils with herbs and balsamic vinegar 101
Open avocado and tomato sandwiches 131
Pan-fried fresh goat's cheese with roast tomatoes and garlic 113
Roasted aubergine, tomatoes and pesto in a baguette 115
Roasted peppers with melted cheese 151
Roasted tomato tarts with salsa verde and wild rocket 154
Rocket and beef salad with a horseradish dressing 139
Scallops with mango and shallot 158
Soft eggs with tomatoes and watercress 137
Spaghetti with marinated tomatoes, fresh basil and garlic crumbs 108
Spicy guacamole with roasted vegetables 117
Spicy vegetable juice cocktail 44
Thai grilled-beef salad 145
Tomato puff with pesto and olives 104
Tomato salad with cucumbers, feta cheese, oregano and mint 97
Tomato sauce for pasta 107
Tomato soup with garlic and lots of herbs 83
Tomato and watercress salad with hazelnut dressing 92
Tomatoes with chives 132
Tomatoes with fresh basil and Parmesan 94
Warm tomato scones 129
Warm vegetable salad 86
toppings
for bread 119
for muesli or porridge: Warm apricots with ginger 52
for toast: Berry toasts 50
tortillas: Avocado relish with grilled vegetables and salsa in warm tortillas 152
toxins 8, 9
tuna
Fresh tuna Niçoise 87
Japanese style tuna with sweet and hot cucumber 146

ulcers, stomach 7

vegetables 4, 7, 8, 9, 11, 12, 20, 21, 24, **31-2**
British Food Calendar 26, 27
organic 20, 21
'seed' 21
Vegetarian sushi 105
vinegars 29
vitamins 1, 3, 4, 11, 15, **16-18**, 20, 21, 23, 37, 62, 63, 77

walnuts
Muesli – Bircher style 51
Pear, fennel and walnut salad 98
Warm apricots with ginger 52
Warm berry and currant salad 65
Warm tomato scones 129
wasabi 30
Japanese style tuna with sweet and hot cucumber 146
Sashimi salmon, sushi rice and toasted nori 147
water 3, 6, **14**, 19, 20, 21, **30**, 38, 63
water chestnuts: Prawns with Thai flavours 151
watercress 119, 135
Fresh green salad with Parmesan crisps 139
Herb chicken skewers with fresh leaves dressed in oil and lime 142
Lemon and paprika roast chicken with watercress sauce 141
New potato salad 90
Salmon with lime and yogurt 131
Sardines with watercress 111
Soft eggs with tomatoes and watercress 137
Tomato and watercress salad with hazelnut dressing 92
Watercress, orange and fennel 93
Watercress and potato soup 78
Watercress with red chilli and basil 99
watermelon 33, 62
wheat germ 29
Granola 53
Spiced muesli 52
whole foods 20
Wild mushroom stew with fresh herb mash 155
Wild rice salad with tangerines and pine nuts 101
wine 7, 30
Hot fruit compôte with vanilla yogurt 47
Salmon with herb crust and red wine sauce, served with broccoli and Puy lentils 148
Strawberry soup 47

yogurt 21, 37, 38, 62
Avocado with yogurt, lime and red onions 116
Beetroot and yogurt 125
Berry and apple sundae 67
Blackcurrant purée with yogurt 49
Hot fruit compôte with vanilla yogurt 47
Muesli – Bircher style 51
Salmon with lime and yogurt 131
Strawberry soup 47
Sweet potatoes with yogurt and coriander 156
Tiny pasta with fresh herbs 130

zinc 15-16, 62, 119